RELACTATION

A Guide to Rebuilding Your Milk Supply

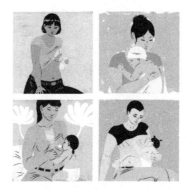

Lucy Ruddle

Praeclarus Press, LLC

www.PraeclarusPress.com

Praeclarus Press, LLC

2504 Sweetgum Lane

Amarillo, Texas 79124 USA

806-367-9950

www.PraeclarusPress.com

DISCLAIMER

The information contained in this publication is advisory only and is not intended to replace sound clinical judgment or individualized patient care. The author disclaims all warranties, whether expressed or implied, including any warranty as the quality, accuracy, safety, or suitability of this information for any particular purpose.

ISBN: 978-1-946665-44-7

Cover Design: Ken Tackett

Developmental Editing: Kathleen Kendall-Tackett

Copyediting: Chris Tackett

Layout & Design: Nelly Murariu

For
Alfie
and
Oliver

TABLE OF CONTENTS

CHAPTER 1

Who Am I and What Entitles Me to Talk About Relactation?

> *"It was the hardest thing I've done and completely worth it."*
>
> ~ Sym, a relactation mum

Hello, and welcome to this book about relactation. To begin, I would like to take some time to share my own story with you.

I have written all of the information in these pages because I am a mother who relactated and because I'm also a mother who had a baby that wouldn't breastfeed. For me, these were two separate babies. However, for many mothers attempting relactation, they are faced with both no milk supply *and* a breast-refusing infant at the beginning of their relactation journey.

Yes, I'm also a peer-supporter, Breastfeeding Counsellor, and an IBCLC, but first and foremost, I am mum to Alfie and Oliver, and it is because of them that I subsequently went on to become any of those things. So, as Alfie and Oliver's mother, here is my breastfeeding story:

Breastfeeding is something I assumed would be pretty straightforward. I mean, how difficult can it be to stick a boob in a baby's mouth eight times a day? Babies sleep a lot, right? So surely I could put my nipple in his mouth for 15 minutes, and then he'd go to sleep in his crib because that is what babies do. I firmly believed this.

Well, as anyone reading this who has had a baby knows, that is all utter nonsense. It's probably not a surprise to learn that I found breastfeeding

REALLY difficult. It hurt—my nipples would burn and sting each time he latched. Alfie cried every time I tried to put him in his crib, but he couldn't be hungry *again* because he just ate two hours ago.

Confused by a reality so different to what I'd been told to expect, I sobbed and cringed my way through a couple of weeks of pain, confusion, and sheer exhaustion before being readmitted to the maternity unit.

There, I found myself surrounded by whispers and mutterings about PND (postnatal depression). You see, I was at significant risk for PND because I had a complicated mental health history. So, when my husband found me weeping on the kitchen floor at 6 am one Sunday and refusing to feed my hungry baby, he called my mother. Together, they looked at me with fear in their eyes and called the midwife, who suggested I come back in "for a little rest."

It's perhaps something of a miracle that I left the hospital 24 hours later, still breastfeeding, but I did. We also had little bottles of formula, because the midwife had said it was more important that I got some sleep, so I didn't end up falling apart on the stone-cold kitchen floor again.

With hindsight, it is no surprise to me at all that within another 24 hours, I was sobbing in the kitchen again. But this time, I decided all this weeping wasn't good for anyone, and I'd just as well stop breastfeeding. My son had received two weeks' worth of my milk, which was more than some babies got. We'd be okay. Formula was fine.

Except what no one really tells you as a new mother is that the desire to breastfeed is often strong, deep, and primal. I could use my logical brain to stop feeding Alfie. I could use it to refuse to express any milk off my sore, engorged breasts. In fact, that bit was easy because my hormone-addled brain told me I'd failed my baby, so I deserved this pain. I could repeat on a loop that formula was easier, just as good, almost the same, fed is best, and happy mummy equals happy baby. Yet, my primal brain wasn't getting the message.

In particular, I hated the warning on the formula tin: "Breastfeeding is best; always consult with a health visitor or midwife before introducing formula." I was hit with shame and guilt every time I put a bottle in Alfie's mouth. The feelings were so intense that I would avoid feeding times and get someone else to feed my baby whenever it was at all possible.

Rather than stopping me from sobbing, this course of action only made me cry more than ever before. I didn't recognise the woman I'd become, and I certainly didn't feel like a mother. Anyone could bottle-feed, but only a mum can breastfeed. I couldn't even get that right.

This went on for two weeks, until one day, I did something that was totally out of character for me. I picked up the phone, and I asked a total stranger for help. The breastfeeding counsellor I spoke to that day told me about relactation, and her words set me off on a path of expressing, skin-to-skin, galactagogues, and eventually, exclusive breastfeeding.

I will never forget the feelings of awe and wonder when Alfie latched to my breast after I'd spent so many days thinking that I had lost our one and only opportunity. I will always remember the first time I had painstakingly collected enough pumped milk over several expressing sessions to put into a bottle to feed him with.

We fell into exclusive breastfeeding one feed at a time, very slowly, over eight weeks, until one day, it hit me that we were actually doing it. For the first time in my life, I had set a goal and seen it through to its conclusion, despite how impossible that goal had seemed at the outset.

Alfie was breastfed until he was 18 months old, and I fell pregnant again. I weaned him at that point because I didn't feel like tandem feeding, which is where you continue to breastfeed your toddler or older child while also breastfeeding your newborn baby. If only I had known how useful a toddler willing and able to remove milk would have been some months later when Oliver was born.

Oliver was what is sometimes called an "aggressive breast refuser," which is to say that he would not latch. In such a situation, many people in our society say, "oh well," and simply formula feed. But, given my experiences with Alfie, I know you'll understand why that was not an option I was up for exploring.

I expressed my milk instead, and gave it to him in a syringe, then a cup, and then a bottle. After some weeks, I stopped battling with him to feed at the breast. I realised I had made things significantly worse by engaging in a daily wrestling match in an effort to force this angry, little creature to feed. He would arch his back, scream, and go puce with rage until I quit the attempt in a haze of my own tears.

This is where my experience of feeding Oliver ties into relactation work. I had to teach him to relax at the breast. We had to recreate the closeness of breastfeeding *without* breastfeeding so that he would feel safe and calm when eventually presented with the opportunity to feed. For weeks, I would feed him with his cheek touching my breast, I would comfort him against my bare skin, practice gentle tongue exercises, experiment with nipple shields, and an at-breast supplementor. (An at-breast supplementor is a tube-feeding device you can tape to your breast. Milk flows from a reservoir, up through the tube, and into the baby's mouth. It can help some babies to go to or stay at the breast for longer, and it can mean that top-ups of expressed milk or formula are given while the baby is breastfeeding, rather than afterwards, thus saving time.)

I carried Oliver in a sling, slept in bed with him (following the Safe Sleep 7 guidance), and made sure he had physical contact with my breast as often as possible. And finally, at 18 weeks old, he latched and fed of his own accord. After that, he was breastfed until he was a little over the age of two.

My experiences led me to train as a Breastfeeding Counsellor, and I quickly learned through my time supporting mums that there was a genuine need for good relactation support. Literature is severely lacking in this area that, with the internet, is a topic that is becoming more talked about than ever. It seems that on every single Facebook or forum post where a mum says she's sad that she's had to stop breastfeeding, someone will almost inevitably chime in with, "Do you know about relactation?"

It seems that both mums and professionals are curious about it. "Is relactation actually possible?" they often ask. And I am here to say, "Yes!"

Not only did I do it, but I have supported countless women to do it as well, both in person and through my Facebook group. I created an online group for people wanting to relactate. It also welcomes those who want to induce lactation for adoptive babies or as part of a same-sex relationship so they can breastfeed the baby their partner or surrogate carried in the womb.

This book is a how-to guide for so many situations: rebuilding a milk supply, building a milk supply from scratch, getting your baby to the breast, or encouraging your child back to the breast after a gap. It can't possibly account for every single unique mum and baby pairing that exists out there, but I do hope that it can give a good, solid foundation for parents as they embark on their own relactation journey. It should also prove useful for professionals such as IBCLCs, breastfeeding support workers, doulas, GPs, and paediatricians who are wanting to find out how to support women and their partners through the relactation process.

At this point, I would like to include a note on my language. I am a white, British mother, and the very nature of my work as an IBCLC in the UK tends to be supporting other white, British mothers. Because of these experiences, the language I use here tends to be female-focused and British. However, I acknowledge, and warmly welcome the wide diversity of parents who find themselves wanting to build or rebuild a milk supply. You are encouraged to substitute any words for your own preferences throughout this text.

It is well documented that here in the UK, we have the lowest breastfeeding rates in the entire world. According to UNICEF, 81% of mothers initiate breastfeeding but by 6 weeks, that number has dropped to 24%, at 3 months, 17% of babies are exclusively breastfed, and by 6 months, only 1% of babies are exclusively breastfed according to the WHO definition (UNICEF UK, Breastfeeding in the UK). We also know that out of the mothers who stop, 80% say they wanted to feed for longer (Fox, McMullen, & Newburn, 2015). That really is a vast number of women who wanted to breastfeed for more time than they managed to. Of course, there are a range of reasons for these dreadfully low breastfeeding rates, and often, it boils down to failing to, or being unable to access good, timely and consistent support.. This systematic review from 2017 states that, "Results of the analyses continue to confirm that all forms of extra support analysed together showed a decrease in cessation of 'any breastfeeding'" (Mcfadden et al., 2017).

Regardless of the cause, women are stopping breastfeeding without realising that they can actually change their minds and try again if they want to. I have supported women to relactate for babies older than 12 months. I have seen babies go to the breast for the first time at a year old. Refugees across the globe are supported through a relactation process as breastmilk is far safer than formula in emergency situations. Relactation is very much an option for those who wish to do it, are well supported, and are given good information to help them on their way.

The question many people ask me is "why?" In a world where formula-feeding is seen as normal, so many people simply do not understand why anyone would want to go through the massive effort that is relactation. As always in matters concerning infant feeding, the answer is not straightforward and is often highly personal to each mother/baby dyad. However, through the time I have spent counselling and supporting mothers online, face to face, and over the phone, a few common themes have emerged:

"My baby is unsettled on formula/has a dairy intolerance/reflux/colic."

There is nothing worse than a miserable baby. Except maybe the niggling doubt that perhaps if you were breastfeeding, they would be happier. From a purely anecdotal standpoint, that may well be right. Mothers often report that babies who struggle with formula seem to thrive on breastmilk, and it's natural to want to offer your baby that opportunity. Many mothers hope that by being able to offer breastmilk, they will have a happier, more settled baby. In fact, donor milk is used across the world for babies who aren't doing well on formula for all sorts of reasons, including Cows' Milk Protein Allergy (CMPA) or intolerance, so we can see that breastmilk works where formula hasn't. Regarding CMPA, Denis et al. (2011) found that 7.5% of babies show signs of CMPA, but that only 0.5% of breastfed babies will develop these symptoms. We can clearly tell from studies like this that breastfeeding protects against CMPA, or at least that because far less cows' milk protein passes through breastmilk than is in formula, that babies simply have less exposure and therefore, show fewer symptoms while breastfeeding.

If your baby has an allergy to something like cows' milk, it's likely (but not a certainty) that you may also need to eliminate that allergen from your own diet. Businco et al. (1999) state that 1ng (one billionth of a gram) of *lactoalbumin* (a protein in cow's milk) needs to be present for the baby to show an allergic response, and that the amount in breastmilk ranges from 0.5 to 32ng/L. It's fascinating that this same study tells us that a single 40ml formula feed contains the same amount of *lactoalbumin* as 21 years of breastfeeding. This is something to be mindful of as you produce more milk. Many mothers say that they notice an improvement in allergy symptoms once their baby is consuming breastmilk, but for some babies, they need mum to cut out dairy products as well. Look carefully at your baby's symptoms in the weeks before you give them your own milk so you can identify whether it's having a good or bad impact once you reintroduce it into their diet. If you do notice an allergen in your diet is causing a problem for your baby, then it's a good idea to talk about an elimination diet with your doctor. What would be even better is if you can persuade them to refer you to a dietician with experience working with breastfeeding babies.

"I miss the connection that I felt while I was breastfeeding."

This is probably the most common reason given to me when I ask mums why they want to relactate. When we breastfeed, we automatically have frequent and often prolonged skin-to-skin contact with our baby's cheek touching our breast. As soon as bottles or other feeding methods are introduced instead, contact between the mum and her baby usually stops. The hormone oxytocin, responsible for the milk-ejection reflex that occurs many times during each breastfeed, helps us to feel connected, bonded, content, calm, and deeply in love. That is not to say that women who only bottle-feed aren't deeply connected with, bonded to, or in love with their babies. It is simply pointing out that a large number of women I speak to report that they notice a change in these feelings when they stop breastfeeding or perhaps, more interestingly, when their baby goes back to the breast for the first time, and they suddenly feel overwhelmed with love and emotion that was lacking before. One lovely case study of 366 mothers talks about how milk production had little to do with how the mothers gauged their success in relactation; they simply wanted the connection that came from nursing their babies again (Auerbach & Avery, 1980).

Babies may feel that renewed closeness too. When a breastfed baby cries, we can offer the warmth and closeness of our breast. When a bottle-fed baby cries, we have to work through a list of jiggling, rocking, nappy-changing, singing, patting, and white noise among other things to try and calm them because their natural need for reassurance and comfort at the breast isn't an option. Often, all that jiggling and rocking takes a lot longer than simply popping a breast in the baby's mouth. We know that breastfeeding reduces pain in infants (Erkul & Efe, 2017), as well as reducing cortisol levels, as they stop crying quickly when given the opportunity to nurse for comfort. It really is a wonderful tool for mothers and babies to use together. It's no wonder that mums say they miss it so much.

"Bottle-feeding is taking too much time/is difficult when we go out and about."

What is particularly interesting about this is that a lot of women will tell me that they stopped breastfeeding because of the time commitment, or because they were worried about breastfeeding their baby while they were out in public. In the first month or so, breastfeeding probably does take more time than bottle-feeding, thanks to newborns needing to feed so frequently, the latch taking time to perfect, and the many growth spurts babies go through. But from around a month on, mums typically report to me that breastfeeding often gradually takes less time while formula-feeding stays the same, or even gets longer as the amount of formula required per feed goes up. Breastfed babies may get more efficient at feeding, and milk supply doesn't keep increasing; it, instead, changes in consistency to meet the baby's changing needs (Neville et al., 1988).

Meanwhile, formula must be given in increasing amounts until solids are introduced because it never changes its nutritional content. We also must factor in washing and sterilising, boiling the kettle, preparing bottles, waiting for milk to cool, and the two hands needed to safely bottle-feed a baby. You can't bottle-feed lying in bed with your eyes closed at 2 am; you must get up, make the bottle, and stay awake while feeding it to the baby. Then the bottle needs washing and sterilising before the next time it's needed.

Going out with bottles is another minefield many aren't aware of until they have no hot water, or forget the powder, or have been delayed for an hour longer than they expected and their baby is screaming for milk that simply isn't available. I'll never forget the story of a mum stranded for several hours in standstill traffic on the motorway who ran out of formula for her hungry, screaming baby. In a wonderful act of human kindness, some local residents got together bottles, water, and powder and the baby was safely fed. But can you imagine the stress and anxiety that poor mum would have been feeling?

In contrast, breasts are portable, the milk never runs out, and it's served at exactly the right temperature with exactly the right amount of water to meet the baby's hydration needs regardless of how hot the weather may be. I noticed the difference in my boys' changing bags when I no longer needed to take bottles of milk and hot water out with me everywhere. In fact, I would often just chuck a diaper and a packet of wipes in my handbag; that was all I needed most of the time once we were feeding successfully at the breast.

"I just really, REALLY wish that I hadn't stopped breastfeeding."

Aside from missing the bonding feelings that breastfeeding brings, this is the next most common reason I hear from mums who are thinking about beginning relactation. Understandably, breastfeeding is an instinctive desire for a lot of women. Our limbic systems don't comprehend that we have access to formula and live in a society where it can be safely prepared. And when breastfeeding ends prematurely, there is often an awful lot of grief, shame, and sense of failure that is felt. Telling mums not to worry, that formula is just as good, that it'll be easier for her now that she can "get her life back," or that now someone else can feed the baby does not help or support her or her baby.

Perhaps she stopped breastfeeding because her doctor gave her incorrect information about a medication. Perhaps her baby had trouble with latching, but she couldn't access good breastfeeding support, and no one helped her to express. Perhaps breastfeeding was painful and a week after she gave up, a tongue-tie was discovered and cut—something that could have made all the difference to her breastfeeding experience.

If you don't have one big reason to relactate, but simply have a sense that you just REALLY want to breastfeed, then congratulations, you are normal. And yes, relactation is possible if you are willing to work hard, and preferably have access to decent support from family, friends, and people who know about breastfeeding and about building up a milk supply.

Guilt

It is important that we pause here and talk a little bit about guilt. When I explore with mums why they want to relactate, guilt, shame, anger, a sense of failure, and low self-esteem often come up. Women, by and large, don't relactate because breastfeeding ended in such a wonderful way that they want to lactate again just for the fun of it. Often, women relactate because stopping breastfeeding was so emotionally traumatic that they are willing to do anything at all to make those feelings stop.

This book (or text) focuses a lot on the practical side of bringing your milk back, but I would urge anyone reading it to think carefully about how they feel regarding the end of their last breastfeeding experience. The burden we carry as mothers is already heavy enough, and we live in a culture that tells us how important breastfeeding is but then lets us down when it comes to actually empowering, educating, and enabling us to do it successfully. There are many books that explore the shortcomings of our society regarding breastfeeding, and there isn't the space to get into it here. However, with background as a breastfeeding counsellor, I would suggest to anyone wanting to embark on this journey to consider what elements of breastfeeding you miss the most. It's quite likely the closeness you felt holding your baby to your breast. This is because breastfeeding is not all about the milk. It is a complete care package for babies and their mothers.

On an instinctive and subconscious level, we know that breast-feeding is so much more than food. A study in 2017 looked at how babies experienced pain during vaccinations (Erkul & Efe, 2017). One group was breastfed during the vaccination, and the other group wasn't. The researchers found that the babies who breastfed had lower heart rates, cried less, and had a higher oxygen saturation level. This all suggests that they didn't feel as much pain as the babies who weren't at the breast while they received their vaccination. What this study doesn't consider is whether it's the act of removing milk, or simply snuggling into a safe adult and suckling that's helping the babies feel less pain. Another study, however, talks about how non-nutritive sucking (where babies aren't actually taking any milk) does seem to also help with pain (Peng et al., 2018). Imagine if we lived in a world where simply allowing your baby to suckle, despite there being no milk in your breast, was acceptable?

Let's also look at this review from 2017 that evaluates whether skin-to-skin contact reduces pain in babies. They conclude that while more study is needed, and there are some limitations to studies of this nature, skin to skin does indeed appear to generally have a positive impact on the pain felt by a baby during a painful procedure (Johnston et al., 2017). The two studies I've discussed here suggest that you don't actually need the milk to support your baby; you simply need skin-to-skin cuddles and access to the breast for suckling.

Finally, I love this quote from La Leche League's *The Womanly Art of Breastfeeding*:

> If you talk to most experienced breastfeeding mothers, they're more likely to focus on the way that breastfeeding helps you and your baby feel connected and attached to each other, weaving an emotional cord to replace the umbilical cord (Wiessinger et al., 2019, p. 10).

Sometimes the process of relactation—the skin-to-skin contact, the extra time with your baby, and the need to find help—can all combine to make the volume of milk unimportant in the end. As we work on the closeness, the value of nurturing comes to the front of our minds. We focus on the calm, warm feeling we experience when our baby's body blends into ours, the steady rise and fall of their breathing, their sweet smell, and suddenly, a full milk supply doesn't feel so essential. Often, this brings with it a sense of peace and of healing, as we learn ways to recreate the closeness of breastfeeding through other means. We can grieve what we feel we have lost and move onto simply loving and enjoying being with our babies.

Interestingly, when this acceptance happens, often that's when relactation suddenly seems to get easier. When we're fuelled by guilt, we can feel desperate and blinkered. We are pumping like crazy, demanding the GP gives Domperidone and scheduling skin-to-skin contact as if it's got to be given X amount of times a day like a pharmaceutical prescription. We're desperate to numb the discomfort of guilt, and we forget what it is that we actually want from having our babies back at the breast, which is usually the closeness.

I would hate for anyone reading this book to get so focused on how many millilitres of milk they can pump that they forget about the rest of the package breastfeeding brings. Don't use relactation as a way to beat yourself up! You have almost certainly done enough beating yourself up already. Your baby wants your warmth and closeness, your eye contact, and your consistent, gentle response far more than he wants breastmilk. And yes, I'm saying that as an IBCLC. This process is about nurturing, not nutrition. As mentioned above, this theory is backed up by a study of over 300 women, who found that it didn't actually matter how "successful" relactation was; it was the act of nurturing their babies with close body contact that felt so important in the end (Auerbach & Avery, 1980).

A Word on Support

I have already mentioned support a few times, so I want to take a moment to talk in more depth about this particular topic that is very close to my heart.

Relactation is a process that requires time and dedication. While it is, of course, possible to do it alone, I would strongly recommend that you seek support from a breastfeeding peer support group, breastfeeding counsellor, La Leche League leader, breastfeeding support worker, or professional assistance from an IBCLC. These people are best placed to understand your desire to breastfeed and to offer encouragement and information as you move through each stage.

My local support group, IBCLC, and breastfeeding counsellor were, quite simply, the reason I successfully breastfed both my children. It's not just me either. Barely a week goes by without someone telling me how their local support got them through various breastfeeding challenges.

It's common for mums to feel anxious about walking into a group or picking up the phone to call a breastfeeding supporter—all sorts of questions may be in your head. This might include, "Will I be judged for not breastfeeding?" and the answer is "absolutely not!" The fact that you are serious enough about relactation to have found a group, or dialled a number, is testament to your dedication, and you will be welcomed warmly.

The power of a listening, knowledgeable, empathic ear should never be underestimated. It is possible that someone you speak to will have successfully relactated themselves, or that the counsellor or group leader will know of someone who has. While it's a fact that mums are far better at knowing what they and their babies need than a breastfeeding counsellor who barely knows them, nevertheless, I would strongly encourage you to seek good local support either before you embark on this journey, or as soon as you possibly can after starting it.

Here are some words from breastfeeding counsellor and peer supporter Laine Perks:

I am both a peer supporter and a breastfeeding counsellor, and I would want mums to know that I, and others in my role, would absolutely want to support mothers if their wish was to relactate. Relactation is about so much more than the milk, and it can be so empowering to know your options when it comes to relactation, and to be able to sit with a mother and help her explore her options is the cornerstone of our support underlined by listening, exploring, and informing. If you're curious, I encourage you to reach out and start that conversation. We would always be there with an open ear, an open heart, and a cuppa!

And some more encouragement from another peer supporter and breastfeeding counsellor, Victoria Mitchell:

As a peer supporter providing face-to-face support at local groups, and a breastfeeding counsellor who takes calls on the National Breastfeeding Helpline, we welcome mums at all stages of their breastfeeding journey who are looking for support and information. A relactation journey often begins with mum being given a safe space to discuss their personal circumstances and experiences surrounding breastfeeding. Exploring their feelings around why and how breastfeeding didn't initially work out as planned, and talking through the reasons for wanting to relactate is just as important as being given the practical information on how to actually go about it.

Peer support can be found with a phone call, via online support groups, or face to face at local groups. All are run by experienced breastfeeding mothers with the desire and training to help others. I've watched the motivation, encouragement, and love given to women through peer support change lives. This seems like a good opportunity to talk a little about the differences in the services. I wrote the following for my blog at the beginning of 2019:

Something that has come up a lot for me over the years of training and experience I've had is this idea that the person at the next level is better at supporting breastfeeding than whatever level I was currently at. As a mum, I idolised peer supporters; as a PS I was desperate to qualify as a breastfeeding counsellor so I could support "better," and the second I passed that qualification, I was nose-deep in IBCLC prep, hoping to become "the best." Now, here I am, an IBCLC, and FINALLY, I see what I've been repeatedly told. There is no hierarchy in breastfeeding support. There is no "better" or "best," only "appropriate for the situation." Let me begin by describing a bit about the different roles you may come across.

Peer Supporters: Training varies across organisations and area, but generally the definition of a peer supporter is a mother who has breastfed for at least 6 months, and who has undergone some training to support mums with common breastfeeding questions and concerns. This training is often several hours over a good few weeks and includes positioning and attachment, how to help or signpost mums with pain, safe sleep, and listening skills. There are also regular training updates.

A peer supporter probably (not always) runs your local breastfeeding group. During an average session, she will welcome all mums warmly, and then help someone to find a comfortable position to feed in, listen to a mum explore her feelings about formula top-ups, chat to someone else about frequent night feeds, make a cup of tea, hand out the biscuits, and tell another mother how to contact the drugs in breastmilk information service.

They extend far beyond group though. You probably have a mate who's a peer supporter or a friend of a friend. She might start a conversation with you at the school gates, or in the play cafe. She doesn't mind if you message her at a weird time of day or on the weekend, because it's likely she's awake breastfeeding as well. She can send you information that's evidence-based on a huge range of problems, and she supports you, cheers you on, and celebrates or commiserates with you throughout your breastfeeding journey.

Peer support is vital to successful breastfeeding in many communities. Mothers have always supported mothers, and peer support takes those mothers and empowers them with a solid foundation in listening and practical skills and knowledge so they can go out into their community to hold up and sit with their fellow mums. Many, many women will say a peer supporter is the reason they successfully breastfed.

Breastfeeding Counsellors: There are several routes to BFC in the UK. Your local counsellor might be trained by the Association of Breastfeeding Mothers, La Leche League, the Breastfeeding Network, or the National Childbirth Trust. They have usually been a peer supporter before going on to BFC. The training varies depending on the charity, some are all remote learning with practise counselling scenarios over the phone, and some have more face-to-face training. However, it's fair to say that a BFC will have listening skills and a lot of education around breastfeeding. They may provide your local antenatal education and may offer home visits. If you call a national breastfeeding helpline, you will speak to someone qualified to the level of BFC.

When you speak to a BFC, you will usually find that what you think is a quick question will become a full, and perhaps lengthy conversation about all sorts of things that you didn't realise were linked. They are called counsellors because they COUNSEL. This means that they actively listen, reflect, share drops of information, use open questions, and careful use of silence to help you work out the answer to your worry or question. They are also skilled at positioning and attachment, self-help for an array of breastfeeding concerns (alongside appropriate medical support where necessary), and can hold a safe space when breastfeeding ends.

IBCLC: An IBCLC is a member of the healthcare team and provides clinical support for breastfeeding. They are very experienced and qualified; many of them came from peer support or BFC backgrounds before they went on to undertake an additional 90 hours of education and sit the IBLCE exam. Often dealing with complex or unusual cases, an IBCLC may be able to help if no one else has quite got to the bottom of your worries. Of course, IBCLCs in private practice can (and are happy to) support families with common worries as well. But if I consider the last five consultations I've had, three of them didn't require specific IBCLC skills; a BFC or PS could have supported them instead if the parents preferred. IBCLCs are well placed to help you if you want to see one person, in the comfort of your home, safe in the knowledge that they are absolutely, appropriately qualified, much how you might hire a private midwife.

So now I've laid out the differences, I hope you can already see how the roles overlap. A good IBCLC will use listening skills just like a PS or BFC. They will back up their recommendations with the same evidence you could get from your PS or by calling a helpline. The differences are far more subtle, and it's not about someone being "better" qualified than someone else.

Imagine you have a headache that won't quit. The first thing you may do is see your GP. They'll give you some suggestions, maybe prescribe you some painkillers, and ask you to come back in a week or two. If your headache still doesn't go, they might refer you to a neurologist who will do more in-depth work to find the cause of your pain. They might refer you to a pain clinic. The GP, neurologist, and the therapist at the pain clinic are all highly qualified individuals in their particular area of medicine.

Breastfeeding support is similar. A peer supporter is going to be an expert at putting you at ease, sharing info, tweaking a painful latch, knowing who else is available locally for specific support, and empowering the vast majority of women to breastfeed. The BFC will be excellent at unravelling your less obvious fears, as well as giving you a bit more, or slightly different info. The IBCLC will be able to home in on your specific situation and use clinical skills to back them up. No one is doing a better job than the other, but everyone knows their boundaries and remit, and will send you to the next person when those limitations are reached, just like the GP.

So, if you're seeking support, think about what you want. If you would like to make friends, have someone bring you a hot drink, be with other breastfeeding mums, or if you're just beginning to experience problems, you're not sure what support you need, or your worries are more niggling doubts. If you think your worry is common (pain, sleep, questions about supply, for example), then pop into your nearest support group. Chances are a PS can help and, if they can't, then they will know where to signpost you next.

If getting to a group isn't possible, you're anxious, or away from home, if a problem is ongoing or overwhelming, you have lots of feelings to begin unpacking, or peer support hasn't quite helped, then call a helpline or find your local BFC.

If you want to pay for consistent one-to-one support in your home, or have complex issues, then you might want to look into IBCLC support.

None of these are mutually exclusive; when I see some-one as an IBCLC, I always encourage them to go to their peer support group. When I'm on the helpline, I might sometimes suggest the mum find a local IBCLC, as well as speaking to us. As a peer supporter, I often give out helpline details for mums to get additional support away from the group. Breastfeeding supporters are a team, we work together, refer to each other, share knowledge, and we all use our skills to support you on your breastfeeding journey.

The above article from my blog touches on IBCLC support alongside the free services you can access across the UK. An IBCLC usually charges for their work, although you can find them volunteering in some locations, and some do work for the NHS. Below are a few words from a fellow IBCLC, Emma Pickett, talking about how a lactation consultant can support you if seeking one is a route you would like to consider:

When you hire a lactation consultant, you have someone who can devote time to your situation and goals. You aren't grabbing 20 minutes in a busy drop-in but sitting down with someone who can give you 90 minutes of their time and more. They can talk you through why breastfeeding may not have gone smoothly from the beginning. Their technical knowledge and experience of breastfeeding problems means they can really help you to investigate what might have happened first time round if you aren't sure.

There may be problems still to resolve, however hard you work to re-build your supply. They can help you develop a plan to rebuild supply and to restart breast-feeding. They know about pumps and what has worked for others and help you make a plan that works for you and your family. It can take time for a baby to re-latch, and you may need to try some positions you haven't used before. Doing that alongside a lactation consultant who can help guide you can make all the difference. Lactation consultants may not have all the answers, but we usually know how to find them. And our passion and dedication for breastfeeding means we absolutely get why this matters. We are never going to say, "Is this worth it?" If you feel it is, we are alongside you.

The other element of support that I ask you to consider is in relation to the practical day-to-day stuff. If you have a partner, are they on board with you relactating? Have you even spoken with them about it yet? If not, you need to have that conversation. Having someone to wash bottles, hold a crying baby, look after older children while you express, and basically look after you is incredibly helpful for so many mums.

If there isn't a partner, how about another family member or a friend? I know many of us can be a bit weird about asking for help in the UK, but in general, people will only agree to do something if they want to. Think about who can bring you some food, push your vacuum around, or do some laundry for you. The sort of support you were probably encouraged to seek out when your baby was a newborn. Making a new milk supply is hard, time-consuming work. It is going to be an awful lot easier if you have a whole team of helpers around you, especially ones who tell you how amazing you are and bring you cake on a regular basis. Cake, along with tea, can make pretty much anything feel better, I believe.

You may also want to consider hiring a postnatal doula to come in and support you. A doula is someone who supports mothers, families, and babies throughout the childbearing year, and often beyond. It's not uncommon for doulas to be asked to support families after their baby is over the newborn stage, and many are happy to do so. While a birth doula would help prepare you for labour, be with you alongside your midwife and partner when the time comes, offering things like massage and affirmations, as well as advocating for you and your needs to the professionals in the room, a postnatal doula will come in after birth and help you to adjust to life with a newborn. Part of this in the case of relactation may be helping you get set up with the breast pump, holding the baby, preparing you nutritious meals, and emotional support. You can find a doula through Doula UK (doula.org. uk) or by asking in your local community. There are a good number dotted around now. They do charge for their work, but Doula UK offers a fund to support those who may not be able to afford a doula, and they also offer vouchers on their website that family and friends could purchase for you if they want to know how they could help. As far as I'm concerned, doulas are truly worth their weight in gold.

Here are some words from Maddie McMahon, a doula trainer and author. Maddie's website is well worth a visit, too (www.developingdoulas.co.uk).

> The word doula may seem newfangled, but the concept of mothers being supported by other women is as old as the hills. One way to describe a doula is "well-informed friend"; rather than telling you what to do, the magic of the doula is to be both a sounding board and a signpost. By providing non-judgemental support and unconditional positive regard, we build a mother's sense of autonomy and self-esteem. And by signposting and suggesting people and services that may be beneficial, we ensure parents have access to all the information and choices that can smooth their journey through the rollercoaster ride of new parenthood. Doulas are not experts and should never, ever tell you what to do; but like Sherpas, we have walked this path before and may be able to point out potholes in the road and walk by your side as you navigate crossroads in your journey. Oh, and we make a mean cuppa.

The Opinions of Family and Friends

Talking about the people around you, relactation is sometimes difficult for friends and family to get their heads around. You may be met with anything from confusion to outright hostility when you tell those closest to you what you plan to do.

This is most likely linked to a concern for your wellbeing, especially if these people who love you so much have already watched you breastfeed, feeling helpless as you struggled to once before. They may be worried that putting yourself through trying to breastfeed once again will be detrimental to your mental health and your wellbeing. It's essential to acknowledge those concerns. They come from a place of love because your nearest and dearest naturally want to protect you. In addition, breastfeeding is so poorly understood in our culture that they may not be able to see any positive outcome to your attempt. The other reason for initially unsupportive reactions is often that people really don't understand the value of breastmilk in our society. They may genuinely not understand why you would want to go to so much effort to provide your own milk to your baby, especially if the baby seems to be doing well on formula.

In these situations, many mums report that the most helpful way to handle it is simply to acknowledge everyone's concerns, then tell them how important it is to you to try, that you want to do it, and that you hope your family and friends will support you to work towards your goal. It might help to have some facts ready to dish out, like how, according to The Iowa Extension Service, just a teaspoon of breastmilk contains 3,000,000 antibodies to protect your baby from illnesses (Bonyata, n.d-a).

You may also decide to be selective regarding who you confide in about your goal to relactate, at least at the beginning. It's often far better to have a couple of supportive people onboard, like a partner and a close friend, rather than your entire friendship circle. You might find yourself dealing with endless questions and possibly even defensiveness from those around you who had a difficult breastfeeding experience and moved to formula.

I found it interesting how some formula-feeding mothers in my wider circle reacted quite strongly to me talking about my relactation journey. Sadness, anger, and often guilt would come up for them, so be prepared and remember these reactions reflect a society where a huge importance is put on breastfeeding while at the same time, the support needed simply isn't provided, and women are being failed. I'd certainly be angry at that, wouldn't you?

Studies back up this idea that many mothers feel anger, guilt, or shame regarding their breastfeeding experiences. A 2019 Australian qualitative study noted that the women interviewed described feeling "devastated" at stopping breastfeeding before they wanted to (Ayton et al., 2019).

CHAPTER 2

Getting Started

> "Relactation is a marathon, not a sprint. It is
> a long, hard journey but the prize at the end
> is worth every tear. So, cut yourself some slack
> because even trying makes you a superhero."
>
> ~ Sym

Relactation is essentially a three-part process:

1. Rebuild a milk supply.

2. Teach the baby to feel comfortable enough at the breast to feed effectively.

3. Establish feeding at the breast.

I will discuss each in turn, but you will most likely need to work on rebuilding a milk supply and building the baby's comfort at the breast at the same time. It's quite likely that one will prove to be more challenging than the other. Some mums easily rebuild a full milk supply but find that their baby fights aggressively at the breast and won't latch, while other mothers have babies who are happy to latch but then they struggle to produce much milk. Some lucky mums have no major challenges at all, while some unfortunate mums find that everything is a battle right off. All of this is normal, all of it is okay, and all of the above can be improved or completely resolved with patience and time.

View this process as a marathon, and not as a sprint. You may well find yourself going backwards and forwards for weeks, feeling like you're getting nowhere at all, and wondering why on earth you're even bothering. This is a common theme, but knowledge is power. Knowing you may need to be best friends with a breast pump for several months is far less stressful than expecting to be fully breastfeeding after a week, which is also possible, by the way. Having seen many mums go through the relactation process, a good guide for how long it will take to re-establish your milk supply is related to the amount time for which you haven't been feeding. So, if you stopped breastfeeding three weeks ago, it may take around three weeks to get back to it. Research is woefully lacking in this area, so I can only talk about my own experiences supporting relactation and talking to those who have achieved it.

First things first, though: we need to talk about breast pumps. While relactation is technically possible without a pump, most people seem to agree that once milk is beginning to be produced, it is much quicker and easier with one. In the relactation group on Facebook, we have seen only one or two mums relactate with hand expression, compared to dozens who reported that they prefer to use a pump. Ideally, you want to look for a double-electric breast pump. If it's marketed as "hospital grade," then that is even better. You're going to be expressing both breasts every two to three hours for around 15 to 20 minutes. If you can do both at the same time, then you're clearly going to be done 15 to 20 minutes sooner.

You can buy double breast pumps online, or in some of the larger baby shops. You can also hire them from a Sure Start Children's Centre if you're fortunate enough to still have one nearby. Ardo is a WHO code-compliant breast pump company that offers next-day delivery on their pumps for hire. However, you may find it cheaper to buy one if you're planning on using a pump for more than a few weeks.

How Much?

The cost of a breast pump can be off-putting at first glance, and one thing to weigh up is the cost in formula and bottles if you don't relactate. The All Party Parliamentary Group on Infant Feeding and Inequalities (APPG) commissioned First Steps Nutrition to complete an inquiry into the cost of infant formula in the UK in 2018. They responded with a range of £6.44 to £32.20 per week, with the most common brands coming in at £13.52 and £8.37 per week, just on the formula (without taking into account the bottles, teats, electric and water costs, and sterilising) (First Steps Nutrition, 2018).

A decent breast pump can be bought for around £100. You might be tempted to buy a second-hand pump, which many mums wonder about. There are a few things to consider here, as well.

Firstly, there is a theoretical risk of contamination. The U.S. Food and Drug Administration (FDA) is clear on its stance that breast pumps are single-use items that shouldn't be passed along because of the risk of contamination (FDA, 2018). While it is possible to minimise this risk by buying a pump that has a "closed system" (a valve in the top of the bottle that prevents milk flowing into the tubing), it is not possible to totally guarantee the complete safety of milk expressed with a single-user pump used by someone else.

Secondly, breast pumps wear out very slowly, becoming quietly less and less effective as time goes on. It can be difficult to gauge whether the preloved pump you bought is nearing the end of its life by simply using it. You could pump for weeks and see no improvement in supply simply because your pump wasn't doing what it's supposed to do without you knowing it.

Thirdly, unless you have bought the pump from someone who you know and trust, there is a possibility that it may have been stolen. I have known of pumps being stolen from children's centres and being sold online; something that's especially easy to do in a world where eBay exists.

Pumping

So, you've got your pump. Now what? Well, you need to think about how milk production works. In summary, the breast is stimulated by a baby, pump, or hand, which sends a message to your brain, saying that milk is needed. It's like buying something online; the pump is you clicking "buy now," and your brain is the company receiving your order and packaging it for delivery (Wambach & Riordan, 2016).

Breastfeeding works on a simple premise: you need to remove milk to make more milk. We need to trick your body into thinking that lots of milk is needed, so it steps up its game and increases production. To do this, we try to mimic a newborn baby. The average newborn feeds 8-10 times per day (or more). It's widely accepted that pumping at least 8 times a day yields the quickest and most significant results when relactating. This is because it's what we do to build and maintain a supply for a non-latching newborn, and it's the minimum number of times a baby should be feeding at the breast. So, get set for a LOT of pumping (Wambach & Riordan, 2016)!

At least one of your sessions should be at night (between 1 am, and 3 am). You should try to go no more than 2-3 hours between sessions during the day and about 6 hours at night. This study discovered that milk production would slow down if mums were going longer than 7 hours without pumping (Lai et al., 2019). However, bear in mind that we count time from beginning of a pumping session to the beginning of the next pumping session. Plus, you need to get into bed and go to sleep.

For example, your sessions might look something like this:

6 am

8 am

10 am

12 pm

3 pm

6 pm

9 pm

3 am

6 am

Or this:

6 am

9 am

11 am

2 pm

5 pm

7 pm

10 pm

1 am

6 am

Most lactation professionals believe that it's absolutely fine for mums to have a 5-6 hour break overnight if they're pumping. There are references to this in many published books and articles on the topic, including *Breastfeeding Made Simple* by Nancy Mohrbacher and Kathy Kendall-Tackett, and *Breastfeeding and Human Lactation* by Karen Wambach and Jan Riordan.

Prolactin

Why pump in the middle of the night? It has to do with prolactin. Prolactin is the hormone responsible for telling your body to make milk. It has a circadian rhythm and is highest in the early hours of the morning (Madden et al., 1978; Wambach & Riordan, 2016). So, if you stimulate your breasts when prolactin is highest, you're sending a strong message to your body to hurry up and make more milk, please.

This same logic is also behind why pumping every 2-3 hours is important. Prolactin levels double when you stimulate your breasts and reach their peak about 45 minutes after the beginning of a feed or pumping session (Noel et al., 1974). We want to raise those levels as often as possible; eight or more pumping sessions a day means that prolactin hasn't declined completely before the next session. Cox et al. (1996) discuss how more than 8 breastfeeds per 24 hours stops prolactin levels dropping before the next feed. We can apply this to breast stimulation with a pump or your hands.

We also know that frequent, effective removal of milk speeds up milk production, whereas allowing milk to build up in your breasts slows production as a whey hormone called Feedback Inhibitor of Lactation (FIL) (Cregan & Hartmann, 1999) increases and tells your body to make less milk because it isn't needed. Your body doesn't like waste, so if milk isn't removed, then it makes sense for your body to conserve energy by making less milk.

To put it simply: raised prolactin levels plus frequent, effective, and thorough milk removal equals more milk, quicker. As a result, prolactin levels remain high, and we can avoid full breasts by frequently stimulating them.

Something else that helps raise prolactin levels is double pumping, which is good news because double pumping is, as discussed above, much quicker than single pumping, and is more effective as well. Auerbach (1990) found that three out of four mothers pumped more milk if they double pumped, compared to single pumping.

Pumping Know-How

So far, you have learned that you need to:

- » Pump 8 times a day, at least once overnight.
- » Pump for around 15 minutes each session.
- » Express both breasts each time you pump.

There are more technical details to this pumping business, though.

To start with, let's do some expectation management. What are you going to see in those bottles? The answer is perhaps nothing, at least initially. If you've had a long gap in breastfeeding, then your breasts may have completed what's called "involution" (where you completely stop making milk). In this case, it's going to take a while for them to get back into the swing of things. However, if you only stopped breastfeeding a week ago, chances are that you're still waking up in a puddle of milk in the mornings and you may be surprised to find milk coating the bottom of the bottles, or even enough to measure in MLs. The more milk you have, the more likely it is that you will see a quicker increase.

My own experience was that once it started to increase, it doubled every few days until reaching a peak after about three weeks. Everyone's experience is different, though. Some people express nothing more than drops for weeks and then suddenly notice it increasing just as they're ready to give up. There is no normal here, no expectation. Your body is totally unique, just like your breasts and milk are totally unique as well. We simply must take this one pumping session and one day at a time.

Now, on to the practical bits. We are fortunate enough to have a range of techniques to use, which help us to express more effectively. A toolbox of resources, if you like.

Flange Size

The flange is the funnel that you place over your breast. You may not be aware that they come in different sizes to fit a wide range of nipples.

If your flange is too small, your nipple will rub against it, causing pain and a red ring around the base, or even vasospasm of your nipple when you take your breast out at the end of the session.

If the flange is too big, it will draw too much breast tissue into it, and that will also cause pain. Both issues reduce milk flow and risk some pretty nasty damage to the breast. You want to look for a flange that allows the nipple just enough room to slide in and out without rubbing. You want something that is a close fit but not snug.

Pump Settings

Your pump likely has a huge range of suction strength and cycle speeds. It's tempting to turn both up to the highest setting and grit your teeth as your nipple is nearly pulled off your breast. However, we know this doesn't help.

Let's go back to a breastfeeding newborn. The first minute or so of a feed, they will do fast, light sucks to trigger a let-down of milk. Once the milk starts to flow, they slow down their sucking as they swallow more often. We can try to mimic this with the pump (World Health Organization, 2009).

To begin with, turn the suction down low and the speed up high until your milk starts to flow. At that point, turn down the speed and increase the suction. Mums often ask how high the suction needs to be, and the answer is the highest setting that feels comfortable. We want to avoid pain because pain will inhibit oxytocin release and therefore, milk flow. The impact of stress and pain on letdown was first talked about all the way back in 1948 (Newton), and in 1994, Ueda et al. found that pain reduced the number of oxytocin pulses, and therefore, the mother's letdown reflex (Wambach & Riordan, 2016).

Pain may also lead to damaged nipples and a miserable time expressing. Try to avoid the temptation to keep turning the suction up because you think it will draw out more milk; it simply will not work.

Warm Compresses and Massage

Before you even get the pump on your breasts, it's a good idea to start by using your hands and warmth to get things started. Some mums ask why they should make pumping take even longer than it already does with massage and heat.

Think about a newborn baby placed skin-to-skin near the mum's breasts. What does he do? He wiggles and squirms his warm body to a breast and begins to nuzzle the nipple with his mouth and nose. He pats, kneads, and rubs the breast with his hand (Matthiesen et al., 2001; Widsrom et al., 1990).

This is the beginning of breastfeeding. He's announcing his arrival to your breasts. Your nipple becomes erect, and oxytocin starts to flow. What does oxytocin do? It makes the milk ducts contract to squeeze out the milk (Leake et al., 1981).

Now think about your breast pump. It's cold and mechanical. It isn't cute to look at, and it certainly isn't going to prepare your body to release milk. However, a nice, warm flannel combined with some gentle massages and nipple rolling from your own hands can go some way to replacing your baby's messages that it's time to release the milk. You only need to do this for a few minutes; it doesn't need to become a massive pre-pumping ritual that feels tedious.

Hands-On Pumping

Jane Morton and her colleagues at Stanford University (2009) are responsible for coining the term "hands-on pumping." In her work, she describes how mothers who use this technique can nearly always yield noticeably more milk than those who don't. The logic to this seems to work along the same lines as massage and heat before expressing (mentioned above), as it's much more like having a baby at the breast.

Babies will often squeeze, pat, and even hit their mother's breasts while feeding. Many lactation professionals believe that these are actually built-in reflexes to get more milk out, like a kitten kneading its mother's breast tissue with its paws. We can recreate that with hands-on pumping.

According to Jane Morton's work, while expressing, you should use your hand to massage as much of the breast as you can. When the flow stops, you should compress the breast to see if you can squeeze out some more milk. Often, this even elicits another let-down (when the milk forcibly pours out of your breast).

How should you compress? It's pretty simple; make a C-shape with your index and middle fingers under your breast, with your thumb on top. Try to have your hand far back, nearer your chest wall than the pump flange or the baby's face. Then, simply squeeze firmly but not painfully and hold that squeeze. If pumping, you should see the milk start to drip or flow again. If feeding, you should see the baby swallowing again. You could also use the heel of your hand. Simply push into the breast and hold, as with the C position.

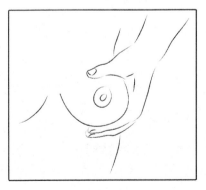 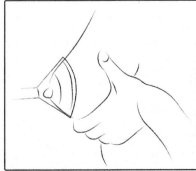

If nothing happens, try another place on your breast, perhaps a bit higher, a bit lower, a bit to the left or the right. Play around and see if you can hit a "sweet spot," where you locate a nice, full duct just waiting for a compression to get it flowing.

Hand Expression

Hand expression is often overlooked, but it can be a great way to end a pumping session. Alternatively, it can be used in the very first days of relactation when your supply is especially low. There are benefits to hand expression as well, namely that it is free and entirely portable. Hand expression can take a few attempts to learn, but once you've cracked it, it can really help you to feel more confident and familiar with your breasts, and, as already mentioned, you can do it anywhere so if you find yourself in a pinch with no pump, being able to hand express instead could be hugely helpful to you.

Jane Morton (2010) at Stanford University suggests the following method, which is also found in Alyssa Schnell's *Breastfeeding Without Birthing.*

Place your thumb and forefinger around the breast, about one inch behind the base of your nipple and press, compress, and release.

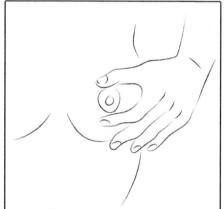

1. Press the fingers towards your chest wall, but don't pull the skin.

2. Compress your fingers towards each other.

3. Release the fingers.

4. Repeat.

There are many videos on YouTube demonstrating hand expression.

Your hands can work on individual ducts, whereas a pump can only create a vacuum and pull the milk out. Five minutes of hand expression at the end of a session can yield promising results, especially when every drop counts in the early days of relactation. This milk is often the highest in fat too, making it incredibly beneficial to give to your baby. One study states that "hindmilk" (the milk that is more readily available at the end of a breastfeed) contains 2-3 times higher concentrations of fat compared to milk at the start of a feed (Ballard & Morrow, 2013).

You might even find that the first few times you express you want to skip the pump altogether. Precious drops can be lost in the machine, but if the milk is hand expressed onto a teaspoon or into a 1 ml or 5 ml syringe, it can be fed directly to your baby, even if there's hardly any milk at all.

Even tiny amounts of breastmilk have been shown to be beneficial for babies, so don't be disheartened by your droplets. A randomised controlled trial in 2008 looked at IQ scores of babies exclusively breastfed, partially breastfed, and not breastfed, and they found that even babies partially breastfed had higher scores than their exclusively formula-fed peers. They found that the more breastfeeding, the higher the IQ scores (Kramer et al., 2008).

A meta-analysis in 2011 also discussed how any breastfeeding increases protection against sudden infant death syndrome, with more protection again in exclusively breastfed babies (Hauck et al., 2011).

Both of these studies show how even a little bit of breastfeeding helps to improve outcomes for babies, so yes, your tiny drops of milk really make a difference.

Start or Finish with the Baby at the Breast

If your baby is willing (which we will discuss later), you can begin or end your expressing session by offering your breast. That can really boost production. All the massage, pumping, and compressing in the world will never send as strong a message to your body as an actual, real-life baby who is able to latch and suckle well.

The key here, though, is a *willing* baby. We do not want to make your breast a stressful place to be. If your baby cries, protests, or refuses to latch, then don't push it. This particular tool is not essential and *must* be baby-led. If you have a baby who cries, pushes away, arches, and refuses to latch, you will need to leave this section until she is happy to latch. Chapter 5 explores how to get to that stage.

In the early days, hand expressing for 15 minutes is a fantastic aim. Precious drops of milk can be lost in the tubing of a pump and are often harder to come by with a pump to start with. As your milk begins to flow again though, you will probably find a breast pump more effective, and you might want to think about changing it up. Do see what seems to work best for you, though; some women simply don't respond as well to a pump as they do with hand expression. If this is you, it's totally fine to only hand express.

After 15 minutes, if milk is still flowing, then keep going. Wait for it to stop but avoid pumping for more than 30 minutes because sore nipples are not fun, and there's no evidence it does any good. Waiting for the flow to stop ensures that you have removed as much milk as possible. This will tell your body that you need even more to be made, and it will respond.

TENS Unit

I just want to squeeze in a little bit about using a TENS unit in the early days of relactation. It was only towards the end of writing this booklet that mums in my Facebook group brought this idea to my attention.

A TENS unit uses a tiny electrical current that moves from one electrode to another on a channel. These currents stimulate the nerves that they come into contact with. The theory is that if we stimulate the nerves around the areola, then prolactin will be released, thus helping your body begin to make milk. However, it is important to note that you should **not** use a TENS unit if you have a pacemaker, and you must never cross channels over your heart.

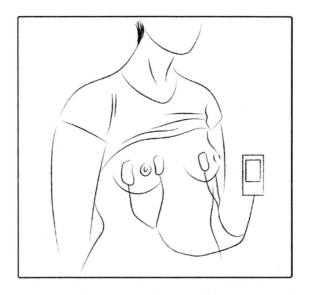

I have attempted to find scientific evidence to support this interesting theory, and have (surprise, surprise, given that this is a niche area of breastfeeding) found nothing evidence-based. Anecdotally, however, there are many accounts on the internet of women who say they believe it helped.

Here's how to use one:

» You place both wires from the same channel on one breast. Position them on either side of your nipple, about an inch away. You should have a straight line crossing from left to right of the + pad, your nipple, and the - pad on each breast.

» You want a low amplitude setting with a long pulse and frequency, which mimics a baby suckling, so around 60-70.

» You can either use the unit every couple of hours for the same amount of time you would pump (about 15 minutes), then still pump/hand express as normal before or after using it (incorporating the TENS into your expressing routine) or if you're not going to be able to express because you're out in meetings or driving for example, then you can use the TENS unit to replace those expressing sessions. However, this only works until milk starts to be produced. Once the milk is there, it isn't enough just to stimulate the breasts; you need to remove what's in there in order to get more being made. You can then hide the unit inside your clothes and go about your daily life with no one knowing you are stimulating your breasts the whole time.

I want to reiterate again that there is absolutely no scientific research to back up the use of a TENS unit. Furthermore, if you have any concerns regarding your heart, you would be well advised to stay away, or at least discuss it carefully with your GP first.

This is an area with little understanding, and I would advise you to read up further on it before making a decision.

"The first time you get enough milk to put in a bottle will feel like you've won Gold at the Olympics." - Sym

Pumping Top Tips

Above is the standard information you can expect to be given about how to express in order to yield the most milk and be successful in your mission to relactate. This next section provides more of the day-to-day tips and tricks that may make pumping easier, both emotionally and physically.

Expressing is a real labour of love and can feel tedious, boring, and frustrating. It is also time-consuming. Anything you can do to ease up some of those feelings is, quite frankly, a winner in my eyes.

Invest in Extra Pump Parts

Washing up eight times a day can quickly become a job you dread. By buying an extra set of pump parts, you only have to wash up once both sets are used, instead of every single time. Invest in a third set, and life gets even sweeter.

Get Help

I've already spoken about this, but it's so important that I'm going to say it again.

Pumping takes time. Not only are you bottle-feeding and taking care of a newborn, but you are also acting as if you are breastfeeding (and at some point, you *will* be breastfeeding as well as bottle-feeding and pumping). Two hours a day expressing is not to be dismissed as nothing.

Many of us talk about feeling ashamed or simply being unwilling to reach out for support in our Western culture. But being brave enough to ask for practical help can bring wonderful results. When I posted on Facebook asking for some backup, I was amazed at just how many people offered to come and take my toddler to preschool, bring me a cooked meal, pick up nappies, or hold my baby while I pumped or napped. Every single person was relieved and happy to have a job to do to help me. Plus, they all have since told me that they genuinely enjoyed it.

Helping others gives people a warm glow. If there is someone you can ask to do a particular thing for you, then ask them.

Find Something You Can Do While Pumping

Try to keep your mind away from counting those drops of milk collecting in the bottom of the bottles, an activity that many mothers will agree can quickly drive you insane.

It might be a TV series that's exactly the right length for a pumping session, or a podcast or an audiobook. Perhaps it's guided meditation on YouTube or speaking to a friend on a hands-free set. You might be able to pump with one hand free.

I found that once set up, I could hold both bottles by bringing my arm across both of them to keep them in place. By the time I was done pumping for my second baby, I had realised that thanks to the "angle of my dangle," I could sit cross-legged with the bottles balanced on and held in place by my knees, giving me both of my hands free to read a book.

Hands-Free Pumping Bra

These are handy, but typically expensive when bought online. They essentially hold the bottles in place for you. If you're resourceful, you can put your battery-powered pump in a rucksack on your back and move around the house as normal, like some kind of pumping Ghostbuster.

Alternatively, you can make your own hands-free bra by buying a cheap sports bra and cutting slits in the right places. Success is variable, but if it works, then you can enjoy the freedom of both hands, something that shouldn't be underestimated.

> *"The pumping bra was a game-changer for us. It meant I could play with my toddler while expressing, which meant I actually managed to sit and pump for a good amount of time!"* - Lucy

Pumping On the Go

If you're a passenger in a car, then its relatively easy to express on the move. Just buy an in-car plug adaptor or use a pump with a battery option.

Having been clocked in standstill traffic expressing as a front seat passenger, you might prefer to use a breastfeeding cover or something else.

You can also use the in-car adaptor if you're driving. Just pull over somewhere safe to pump first. I've heard stories of women pumping on trains, or in feeding rooms in supermarkets and malls. It's amazing how resourceful we can be for our cause.

Hands-Free Pumps

At the time of editing this book, a particular brand of pump is currently popular with mums, as it's marketed as hands-free. It essentially slips inside your bra and allows you to go about your daily life while the pump does its thing. I have spoken to several clients and to mums on social media about this pump, and have come up with a helpful list of pros and cons, as reported by the pump users:

» You can walk around, cook, sit upright and read a book, have the baby on your lap, etc., while using it.

» You can't lean over very much, as the pump registers the milk container as full when you do and stops. So, you basically need to keep your torso upright while using the pump.

» They can be amazing for pumping on the go—during a dog walk or school run, for example.

» They have lights on them that show through your clothing, giving you glowing breasts.

» Some mums have told me they use the hands-free pump in addition to a traditional one for when they need to get stuff done at home or the baby is fussy. This means that they are more able to fit in pumping sessions they might have otherwise needed to skip.

» The battery life isn't amazing; it will need charging fairly often.

» We don't know how these pumps compare to standard ones for the work of relactation, or for heavy, regular usage. They may not be as effective, and they may not last as long. We simply don't know, as they are so new to the market.

» They are expensive compared to a traditional electric pump.

Keep the Baby Happy

One of the biggest barriers to expressing mothers tell me about is an unhappy baby. Many women find that popping the baby in a bouncy chair facing them, then rocking the chair with her foot while talking and singing will keep the baby happy during the required 15 minutes. Many babies seem to like the white noise of the pump, and along with the gentle bouncing of the mum's foot on the chair, they may even fall asleep.

You might find it helpful to pump while sitting on the floor next to the baby so you can touch her and play with her. Of course, this is exactly where having someone who can hold the baby is perfect. Perhaps you can time some pumping sessions to coincide with friends or family popping by? Or before your partner goes to work, and when they get home again?

Older Siblings

Having pumped exclusively for a newborn, with a 2-year-old also on the scene, I fully appreciate how difficult it can be to entertain both and pump at the same time.

I won't lie; my toddler watched a lot of TV while I pumped, and I ate a *lot* of snacks. It was surprising how quickly pumping became so normal to him that he wasn't interested. I gave him his own pumping set of bottle and flange, and he used to "pum mick for baybee" like Mummy.

I would also set up playdough or colouring for him to do while I pumped next to him at the table. And he loved stickers; my pump was covered by the time it retired!

Occasionally, I did need to abandon a session for one reason or another, but that is perfectly okay. Just pick it back up once everyone is calm again. If you managed six minutes and then had to stop, just do the remaining nine, or another five if you get interrupted again. There will be days like that. It will be okay.

Frequent, short bursts of pumping may even be beneficial to your supply, as we think your body is tricked into thinking a hungry baby is cluster feeding to bring in more milk, which leads me to my next suggestion:

Power Pumping

Power Pumping, or Pumping Boot Camp, is where you express frequently over a short period of time. It generally looks like this:

Pump for your usual 15 minutes.

Take a break for 10 mins.

Pump for 10 mins.

Break for 10.

Pump for 10.

You would do this for one or two sessions a day, for several days, up to a week or even longer if you don't find it to be too much.

I'm not sure who first coined the phrase or the technique; there appears to be no mention of power pumping in academic papers, but it does appear throughout blog posts and articles online, including Kelly Bonyata at kellymom.com, in her article, "I'm not pumping enough milk. What can I do" (Bonyata, n. d.-b)?

Why would you Power Pump? To answer that, consider a cluster-feeding baby. They will feed several times over a block of a few hours, with short gaps in between. This behaviour is a clever way of telling your body that the baby wants more milk. Remember, the more a baby feeds, the more milk is made. The shorter the gaps between feeds, the higher your prolactin remains, and the faster more milk is made. Softer, less full breasts hold milk with a higher fat content.

So, when you Power Pump, you're trying to trick your body into thinking it's dealing with that cluster-feeding newborn. Consequently, it's logical that over time, the breasts may increase production to meet the perceived extra demand. Cluster feeding is discussed across many of the well-respected information books for parents and professionals, including *La Leche League's The Womanly Art of Breastfeeding*, 8th edition (pgs. 107-108), *Breastfeeding Made Simple*, 2nd edition by Nancy Mohrbacher and Kathleen Kendall-Tackett (2010), and *Counselling the Nursing Mother*, 6th edition by Judith Lauwers and Anna Swisher (2015).

> *"In the early days, I had a pumping basket full of nipple creams, snacks, juice cartons/bottles of water, breast pads, etc. so I had everything to hand so I could pump whenever and wherever I needed to. I think it's saved my bacon more than once!"* - Sparkle

Washing and Sterilising

When it comes to washing and sterilising pump parts and bottles, there are endless forum discussions around whether sterilising is essential, and how often to wash your equipment.

You may have read the suggestion that you can simply store pump parts in the refrigerator in a Ziploc bag for up to five days. This is based on the theory that breastmilk is safe in the back of the fridge for this long, so any leftover milk on your pump parts is also safe to be left (NHS, 2016).

However, following a sad case in America where a baby died, the CDC in the States now recommends that pump parts are thoroughly washed in a separate bowl to the family washing-up basin after each use to avoid the risk of pathogens developing and potentially harming the baby (CDC, 2019).

In the UK, the NHS recommends sterilising pumping equipment in between uses, which is easy if you're pumping occasionally but much less straightforward if you are expressing eight times a day (NHS, 2016).

Interestingly, the Academy of Breastfeeding Medicine, which is the authority on this sort of thing over in America, states that washing in hot soapy water and air drying or drying with a paper towel is all that is needed and that sterilising isn't necessary (ABM, 2017.).

One quick method of sterilising, should you prefer the NHS guidelines, is to use a sterilising fluid that you change every 24 hours. You simply submerge your parts in the solution after washing them each time. Check the package instructions, but usually you simply shake off as much excess liquid as you can before using the bottle/ pump parts while still damp from the solution.

There is little concrete information out there about washing and sterilising with regards to breastmilk, though. With formula milk, we know there are pathogens that must be killed with careful cleaning and sterilising after each use. However, breastmilk contains living, useful organisms. It's safe at room temperature for four hours and in the fridge for around five days, unlike formula, which should be used immediately (CDC, n. d.).

One thing that everyone seems clear on is that if you are pumping for a sick or premature baby, then hygiene absolutely must be paramount, and sterilising is essential. You should always wash your hands before expressing and handling the pump parts or milk, regardless of anything else.

Storing and Handling Your Milk

I briefly mentioned milk storage above, so here are clearer guidelines that will be helpful as your supply increases.

You can keep freshly pumped milk at room temperature for 4-6 hours, depending on how warm the room is. This is useful for middle of the night feeds. If you express before you go to bed, and know the baby will wake up in a few hours, then you won't need to worry about warming milk before feeding it. With my non-latching second baby, I used to leave the 11 pm bottle of pumped milk on the kitchen table for my husband to feed our baby at around 2 am, when he woke up for his feed. This 6-hour rule is also incredibly useful if you're pumping while on the go. No need to worry about finding a fridge, as long as you aren't leaving it in a hot car.

If you aren't going to use your milk within the 4-to-6-hour window, then it needs to go at the back of a cold fridge for five days. It's best at the back, where the temperature is most consistent; storing milk in the door means the milk is forever being exposed to different temperatures each time you open it. Some sources suggest six days in the back of the fridge is acceptable, and others, that 3 days is ideal. But five seems to be the standard and most common recommendation.

A frequent question is, "Can I mix milk from different sessions into one bottle?" The answer is yes, as long as both expressions have reached the same temperature first. For example, if you pumped milk at 8 am, and you want to add your milk from 10 am to it, you just need to pop the 10 am milk into the fridge in its container for an hour or two before mixing them into one bottle.

Make sure you use all of the milk in the bottle by the time the oldest reaches day five, however. You can also add milk that is chilled to already frozen milk. You just need to make sure that you have more frozen milk in your bottle or storage bag than you do chilled, liquid milk.

If you want to store milk for longer than five days, or you haven't used milk in the fridge, then you can freeze it. It's best to use milk storage bags or bottles for this.

Milk can be safely frozen for up to 3 months in the icebox of a fridge, up to 6 months in an upright fridge/freezer, or up to 12 months in a deep freeze, although it's worth noting that quality may start to decline after 6 months. Freezing changes milk composition and kills some of the living parts of it. However, it is still considered to be a better choice than formula where it's available (Hanna et al., 2004).

When you come to use it, defrost it slowly in the back of the fridge. If you want to use it quickly, you can run it under a cold tap to defrost, and then a warm (but not hot) tap to warm through for your baby. You must use this milk right away though.

Shake or Swirl?

Mums are often cautioned not to shake their breastmilk to mix it. When stored in a bottle or bag, the fat rises to the top of the milk and needs to be mixed back in before feeding to your baby. The reason mums are cautioned against shaking breastmilk to mix the fat back in is that we know roughly shaking milk changes it. However, unless you are shaking it like you're trying to mix powdered formula, then you don't need to be overly worried.

You can gently tip the bottle over a few times or swirl it around to mix the fat back together with the waterier milk. No need to get anxious about transporting it on a bumpy car ride, or someone forgetting to not shake it.

To feed your milk to your baby, you will probably want to warm it, although there's no harm in giving them cold milk. Some babies won't drink it cold, but it's not harmful to them. You can hold the bottle under a warm tap or stand it in a jug of warm water.

It's often advised to not microwave human milk. Microwaving increases the risk of hotspots, destroys some of the components, and changes the composition of the milk. However, a study from 1996 found that as long as the milk being heated doesn't reach 60 degrees centigrade, then the loss of nutrients and immunoglobulins is "insignificant" (Ovesen et al., 1996).

Remember to wash your hands before you handle your milk, bottles, or pump parts at any time.

It may seem like a lot of space in this book has been devoted to expressing breastmilk, but that's because pumping will make up a huge chunk of your relactation journey. It's also important that you are pumping well, so you are using your time effectively. It would be incredibly frustrating to pump for 15 minutes every three hours to discover after three weeks that you didn't have the suction turned up correctly, or that hands-on pumping might have sped things up considerably.

Expressing is a real labour of love, one that the mothers I have spoken to say is totally worth it.

CHAPTER 3

Increasing Milk Supply

*"With every ounce I give her, the guilt
I suffer for giving up on bf gets less and less."*
~ Shell

For many women, simply pumping often and offering your baby the breast is enough to bring back a full milk supply over time. (This is assuming the baby is happy to latch. There's more information in Chapter 5 for breast-adverse babies.)

However, there are times when mothers want to use "milk-making herbs and medicines," also known as galactagogues. Galactagogue is a word with Greek origins. It translates as "milk" and "leading," because they are substances that promote lactation, often by raising prolactin levels.

I will begin this segment with a disclaimer: the information here is not meant to replace medical advice. I would always recommend you speak to your GP before taking any herbs or medications with the intention of increasing milk supply.

People often assume that because an herb is natural that it is safe. However, herbs can be incredibly potent, so you should always treat them with respect and only use them if you are confident that they are safe, necessary, and effective.

You can also check out the Breastfeeding Network's Drugs in Breastmilk factsheet for galactagogues, which is informative and a great print-out to take to your doctor.

Galactagogues will only work if you are removing milk frequently. They are to be used alongside a lot of pumping and/or breastfeeding, not instead of. All of the hard work we discussed in the previous chapter about pumping still stands. In fact, unless there is an urgent need for your milk to return to full supply quickly, it would be a good idea to spend at least a couple of weeks trying everything else before even thinking about herbal galactagogues (and even longer before considering taking the pharmaceutical ones).

When I started to research for this chapter, I was shocked at how few actual studies there have been on galactagogues. So, many things people claim will increase milk supply have literally no evidence behind them at all. The thing with galactagogues is that they often have a strongly held place in different cultures. Each country and society seem to have its own special foods they give new mums to help milk supply, and then these get handed down over generations with no one questioning how effective they are.

There is also an argument that galactagogues do work because we *think* they work. They have a placebo effect. We know milk flows better when Mum feels relaxed, so if she believes something she has taken will help, then perhaps that alone is enough.

So, if you feel that sprinkling flaxseed on your porridge oats helps your milk supply, then own that belief. As long as you aren't allergic to a food you're eating, and you enjoy it, then it's highly unlikely to do any harm you. Indeed, the psychological effect could potentially be helpful.

Myths About Galactogogues

There is a lot of misinformation about galactagogues, and I hope to address some of the common myths here before moving on to looking at the ones that are backed up with scientific evidence.

"Drink lots of water."

This likely comes from the information we have, which suggests severe dehydration can temporarily decrease milk production. Therefore, many breastfeeding supporters suggest you drink to quench thirst only. There's no need to make a special effort to stay hydrated. Simply follow the principle that if you're thirsty, have a drink. Kelly Bonyata, at kellymom.com, backs this up in her article, "How does a mother's diet affect her milk?" She says:

> It is not necessary to force fluids; drinking to satisfy thirst is sufficient for most mothers. Unless you are severely dehydrated, drinking extra fluids is not beneficial, may cause discomfort, and does not increase milk supply. It is not necessary to drink only water—our bodies can utilise the water from any fluid.
>
> The main message on calories and fluids—Eat when hungry & drink when thirsty (Bonyata, n.d.-b).

"Eat oats."

Oats are a complete protein, nutritious, and often invoke comforting, relaxing memories of childhood. Oxytocin helps milk to flow, and it's released when you feel relaxed. If you think something you are eating is going to make more milk, then you're more likely to relax around your next pumping sessions. This may very well result in more milk in the pumping bottles. Good nutrition is so useful for postnatal mums. It's as though the theory that oats increase supply could be based on an underlying awareness that nutrition is helpful after having a baby.

So, if you enjoy a bowl of porridge or a flapjack, then, by all means, tuck in. Just don't feel you have to eat endless oatmeal for the sake of it, because you don't. If you don't even LIKE oats, then really, there's no evidence to suggest forcing yourself to eat them will help your milk supply.

"Try Goat's Rue."

While there aren't any recent studies that back up its use as a galactagogue, Goat's Rue is popular with mothers wanting to build milk supply. Indeed, Alyssa Schnell discusses the use of Goat's Rue freely in her book *Breastfeeding Without Birthing*, suggesting it as a good way to build breast tissue (2013, pgs. 177-178).

Goat's Rue usually has no side effects, but it can cause low blood sugar (hypoglycemia) in a mum, so if you have any issues with diabetes or blood sugar, then it's a good idea to avoid it.

"You need this recipe for lactation cookies!"

Isn't it fascinating that lactation cookies can be commercially made and sold? Anything to do with milk production, which can also make a tidy profit, should be taken with a pinch of salt. Key ingredients in these are often oats, brewer's yeast, and flaxseed. All of these ingredients are claimed to increase milk production with little to no actual evidence to back up those claims.

Lactation cookies are often packed with sugar to compensate for the bitter brewer's yeast. They're also expensive both to make or buy. As with oats, if you like them, then carry on and enjoy them, but there really is no evidence that they do anything useful to milk supply.

"How about Mother's Milk tea?"

Another commercial product! I'll give the same info as above; there is little to no evidence that they do anything, but if you enjoy them, then they won't hurt.

Food as Galactogogue

Many cultures have a long history of using certain foods to increase milk supply in lactating mothers. With the explosion of online social-media support groups, these foods are becoming talked about more often again.

We call them lactogenic foods, and while there is little evidence to support any of them, they are worth discussing here. If a food that tastes good isn't harmful in lactation, and eating it seems to yield more milk, or makes you feel like you're doing something to help, then there is no reason not to eat it.

Foods considered lactogenic tend to be nutrient-dense whole foods that we should all be eating anyway. It would be ignorant of IBCLCs to turn our noses up at cultural beliefs and personal experiences because we have no evidence something helps. Indeed, if eating a particular food helps you to relax about your milk supply, that alone may be enough to increase oxytocin and result in an extra let-down. The result will be more milk in your pump bottles. The more milk you remove from your breasts, the more will be made.

Below is a list of lactogenic foods and any theories or studies relevant to lactation.

Barley

Traditionally, women were told to drink beer to increase milk supply. It seems to be that this recommendation was based on the hops from barley. In studies on rats, they found that serum prolactin levels increased in rats that were fed beer and it's the high levels of prolactin that help milk to be produced (Clin, 1988).

Of course, we need to be careful with alcohol consumption while breastfeeding or parenting. Many breastfeeding specialists agree that a unit or two of alcohol a couple of times a week is probably fine. But we don't know when drinking becomes problematic. there are far more reasons why excessive drinking while breastfeeding could be problematic than I can get into here.

I suggest you do your own research; La Leche League International (LLLI.org) has a great article online. So do Kellymom.com, and Dr Jack Newman.

Garlic

This has been used in Asian cultures for centuries and is given to postnatal mothers to support their milk production. In 1986, a poor study was conducted with no placebo, blinding, control, or breastfeeding support offered. The researchers gave forty mothers a supplement called lactare, which contained garlic, liquorice, fenugreek, and wild asparagus (all purportedly lactogenic foods). The mothers were supplementing on day five with perceived low milk supply. None were supplementing four days later (Sholapurkar, 1986).

Fennel

One study found fennel may increase milk supply and fat content in goats' milk (Bone & Mills, 2013). No adverse effects have been found in humans. But there is also no evidence that fennel increases milk supply in human lactation either.

Other Foods

Other cultural and historical lactogenic foods include spinach, sweet potato, brown rice, millet, carrots, yam, peas, leafy green veg, raw almonds, avocados, coconut water, onion, ginger, cashew nuts, and oats.

As you can see, all of these are healthy, well-balanced, whole foods, and unless you are allergic to them, or you feel like your baby reacts to them, there is no need to avoid them in your diet during lactation. They *may* help with milk supply either by increasing prolactin levels or by providing you with the psychological effect of feeling like you're giving everything you can to increasing your supply.

Equally though, there is no need to make a special effort to consume any of these foods as we simply don't have the evidence that they do a lot. What we *do* know is that frequent, effective breast stimulation is far more effective at increasing milk supply than anything else you could ever do.

Galactagogues with (Some) Evidence Behind Them

There are some milk makers that seem to actually help. The first ones discussed below you can get from a health food store or online.

Fenugreek

Fenugreek is widely suggested and is often used by women wanting to increase milk supply. The evidence is mixed; some women notice an increase in supply, while for others, it seems to do nothing.

Supply usually increases between 24 and 72 hours after the first dose, although it can take a couple of weeks to have an effect on some mums.

The suggested dose is at least 3,500 mg (up to 7,000 mg) a day. This is usually taken in the form of 2-4 capsules, three times a day. Check the bottle for the amount in each capsule.

It's usually a good idea to start with the lower end of the dosage. Signs that you are taking a high enough dose includes your sweat and urine smelling like maple syrup or sweet curry.

Warnings for Fenugreek

Drugs.com has in-depth information regarding the safety and contraindications for fenugreek (see https://www.drugs.com/mtm/fenugreek.html). Be aware that some babies don't take well to fenugreek in their breastmilk, and may be unsettled or have an upset stomach.

Fenugreek is not suitable if you have diabetes or any other issue with your blood sugar.

Fenugreek is from the pea family so it may not be safe for you if you're allergic to peanuts or chickpeas.

Fenugreek is not recommended if you have any problems with blood clotting or any bleeding disorder.

You need to be wary of using NSAIDs while taking fenugreek.

There is a possible link with spontaneous abortion, so be especially cautious if you have a history of miscarriage.

Fenugreek can cause nausea, vomiting, and diarrhoea in some mums.

Fenugreek may worsen symptoms of asthma in some mums.

There are also some drug interactions to be mindful of, as fenugreek can slow down the absorption of antidiabetic drugs, anticoagulants, and platelet inhibitors.

Some mums use fenugreek long term, and there are no known risks associated with this if you don't fall into any of the risk categories above.

Pharmacist Wendy Jones, who provides the information for the UK Drugs in Breastmilk information service, and has written books on the subject, discusses fenugreek thoroughly in her factsheet on galactagogues, which can be accessed as a PDF online.

Milk Thistle (silymarin)

Milk thistle has been used traditionally for many, many years, especially in Europe and India. There is some research into milk thistle as a galactagogue too. Women were given 420 mg a day for 63 days and reported an increase in milk supply over that seen with a placebo. There were no unwanted side effects reported (Pierro et al., 2008).

Warnings for Milk Thistle

Drugs.com has a good list of risks, considerations, and contraindications (see https://www.drugs.com/mtm/milk-thistle.html).

While side effects seem to be rare, you may experience diarrhoea, nausea, and vomiting.

You should avoid milk thistle if you are allergic to ragweed, daisies, chrysanthemums, or marigolds, as they're from the same family of plants.

You should not take milk thistle if you are taking Dilantin to control seizures, or if you are taking birth control pills, as it can make them less effective.

You also need to be careful if you're taking antipsychotic or anti-anxiety drugs, cancer medication, or blood thinners.

Always tell your GP you are taking milk thistle before using any prescription drugs.

Domperidone

This is a prescription medication used to treat nausea and speed gastric emptying. A useful side effect is that it also increases milk supply well by increasing prolactin levels (Osadchy, Moretti, & Koren, 2012).

It's worth noting that the only studies carried out on domperidone regarding breastfeeding have been on premature babies. No one has studied the efficacy of this drug in older babies or for relactation.

It is also not licensed to be given for relactation or low milk supply, so finding a GP willing to prescribe it can be understandably difficult. Bear in mind that if a GP decides to give a drug for an "off-label" use like this and something goes wrong, they risk huge repercussions that most likely wouldn't be covered by their insurance. The Medicines and Healthcare Products Advisory Board (UK) is clear on their stance that domperidone should only be prescribed for nausea and vomiting, only for the shortest amount of time possible, and at the lowest dose. However, my experience is that many GPs will still prescribe for lactation as a short-term option.

Warnings for Domperidone

There are risks associated with domperidone too, including heart problems, especially once the dose reaches more than 30 mg per day (30 mg per day is usually what is prescribed for increasing milk supply). It's important to point out, however, that the studies that raised the link between domperidone, and heart problems used an elderly sample group, and many of the participants already had health problems. The medicines and healthcare products regulatory agency released a statement in 2014 noting that there is a small increased risk of cardiac episodes when using domperidone in populations over the age of 60, at high dose, and for a prolonged amount of time.

They state that it should only be prescribed for nausea and vomiting and that the lowest dose should be used for the shortest amount of time (gov.uk, 2014).

However, in their report "Domperidone Versus Metoclopramide Self-Reported Side Effects in a Large Sample of Breastfeeding Mothers Who Used These Medications to Increase Milk Production," Thomas W. Hale, Kathleen Kendall-Tackett, and Zhen Cong, discuss how less than 1% of 1,990 mothers taking either domperidone or metoclopramide (the often suggested alternative to domperidone for milk supply) reported cardiac arrhythmias or a racing heart, and mothers taking metoclopramide were over 3 times more likely to report side effects if they were taking metoclopramide. This research shows us that the risk of problems with domperidone are quite small. This isn't to dismiss the risks, of course—it is important you talk with your GP about any prescription medication to make sure its suitable for you. However, this sort of information can be helpful for aiding your doctor in making the best choice with you.

The usual dose is 10 mg, three times a day, for up to 10 days for building milk supply, although you may find it difficult to persuade your GP to prescribe you a course for longer than seven days. This is something that is important to consider, as suddenly stopping domperidone can lead to a crash in milk supply. If your doctor feels unable to prescribe the medication for long enough to include the necessary tapering off, is it worth it? How upsetting would it be to see an increase in milk supply, only for it to vanish again? Please have a proper discussion with your doctor about this before beginning a prescription of domperidone.

You may notice an increase in production as soon as 24 hours after beginning the drug, but it could also take several days for supply to begin to build. If you don't notice any increase within 7 days, it's probably better to stop using it rather than risk the potential problems from continued use.

It's important that once supply has increased, you reduce the medication in stages to protect your milk. Reducing by one tablet around every five days is often suggested. If milk supply starts to drop during this time, then your GP may be willing to prescribe the medication for another week before beginning to reduce it again.

A systematic review (Bazzan, Hofer, & Theall, 2016) found that out of seven herbal and pharmaceutical galactagogues studied, domperidone had the most significant effect on milk production when compared to a placebo group.

Side effects are rare but can include a dry mouth, headache, and stomach cramps. Doses of greater than 30 mg a day may increase the risk of sudden cardiac death and other heart conditions in the mum.

There have been reports of withdrawal symptoms for mums taking domperidone when they stopped taking it. These symptoms include anxiety, insomnia, depression, and panic attacks (Seeman, 2015).

Metoclopramide

This is another prescription medication for which relactation is an off-label use. As with domperidone, you may find your GP is reluctant to prescribe it.

There is mixed information around how effective metoclopramide is for increasing milk supply. Some studies say it's effective but not as much as domperidone, while others find it has no additional benefit to milk supply once breastfeeding techniques have been worked on properly.

There is also a significant risk of depression (regardless of previous history), especially with long-term use. Many lactation consultants advise against its use as the risk of depression is so high in women taking the drug over more than a couple of weeks. You should absolutely avoid this drug if you do have a history with depression.

You may also experience diarrhoea, nausea, sedation, headache, vertigo, restless legs, hair loss, and even seizures. One American study found that of the 32 women they followed using metoclopramide, all of them experienced adverse reactions to the drug (Bazzano et al., 2017).

The recommended dose is 10 mg three times a day for 7-14 days, being tapered off, like domperidone, at one pill every few days to protect milk supply.

Both domperidone and metoclopramide are used with birth control medication to induce lactation in women who are wanting to breastfeed an adopted baby or for same-sex couples both wanting to breastfeed.

Once again, I want to remind you that drugs need to be used with caution. You should ensure that you have the support of a GP and, if possible, an IBCLC.

I also want to remind you that just because herbs are natural, that does not automatically mean that they are safe. Please do your research before embarking on taking anything that claims to increase your milk production.

Anecdotally, there is probably an entire book that could be filled with mums' stories of success with increasing milk supply following the introduction of various, obscure galactagogues. We shouldn't automatically dismiss them as nonsense, but we do need to hold on to the fact that no galactagogue in the world will make a difference if you aren't frequently and effectively stimulating your breasts.

Explore all of your options and research thoroughly before committing to medication.

CHAPTER 4

Feeding Methods

> *"Just when I was ready to quit,*
> *the drops turned into a flow of milk!'*
> *~ Becky*

Chances are that you're bottle-feeding. You may not be, but it's highly likely that you are. This is okay; please don't feel any pressure to run out and buy a cup, or learn how to finger feed.

However, there are a couple of other ways beyond bottle-feeding to get milk into a baby, which may support relactation. The first method is actually done using a bottle.

Paced Bottle-Feeding

"It was so good for our bond for me to really connect with and communicate with my baby during bottle-feeds. He used to look into my eyes, and it just made my heart swell with this insanely intense love." - Bella

When we feed a baby a bottle of milk, we tend to lie them down on their back in the crook of our arm. We then put the bottle in the baby's mouth and leave it there until the baby either drains the bottle or actively turns their head away. Sometimes your baby will do this, and we will put the bottle back in because they haven't taken the prescribed amount on the back of a formula tin.

When a baby has a bottle in their mouth in this way, they have little to no control over how much milk they take, or how quickly that milk flows out of the teat and into their mouth. As a result, bottle-fed babies often appear to guzzle or gulp down milk in a way that looks like they're starving.

Actually, it's quite likely that they are simply trying to keep up with the steady, often fast, flow of milk. This can lead to overfed and windy babies.

It can also result in what is commonly known as "bottle preference" or "nipple confusion." This is where a baby begins to refuse to breastfeed after having bottles. How does this relate to relactation? Well, one of the first things we can do to help a baby relearn how to breastfeed is slow down the flow of milk and give the baby back some control over feeding.

When breastfeeding, the baby takes the breast into his mouth. We don't "stick a boob in" (although, you may hear that phrase quite often in breastfeeding circles). We offer the breast, and your baby takes it or refuses. They then have some time where they are sucking, and nothing much is happening. It can take a couple of minutes for milk to start flowing from a breast. The milk then sprays out in a "let-down" before slowing again, until your baby triggers another let-down by continuing to suckle.

There are some trains of thought that this rhythm of feeding (flowing and stopping, flowing and stopping) helps the baby to regulate his appetite. This does make sense. For example, as adults, we know we eat more food if we rush our meal. If we slow down and take our time, we can feel our belly telling us it's full before we have eaten more than we need.

When the baby is finished, he falls asleep or pulls off the breast. Because we can't see how much milk he has taken, we have to trust that he's taken his fill and is quite happy if he refuses to take the second breast.

Compare that to bottle-feeding: bottle pushed into the mouth, immediate and consistent flow of milk, and the caregiver can force the baby to take extra milk if they're being led by arbitrary instructions about what amounts to give. This can easily result in an overstuffed baby with a bellyache or huge weight gains.

Enter paced bottle-feeding. Here, we try to mimic breastfeeding, at least a little bit. For combination-fed babies, it may help avoid breast refusal (either due to bottle preference or the baby still being full of formula when the mum offers her breast). For babies who are being coaxed back to the breast during relactation, it just begins to gently transition them away from the fast-flowing rate of the bottle they're used to, which can, in turn, help them accept the breast more quickly.

How do we do this? Let's explore that now.

1. Instead of laying your baby back in the crook of your arm, bring her into more of a sitting/leaning-back position. If you can get her, so her face is close to or touching your breast, even better. This will add to the message that the breast is a good, comforting, happy place to be because there's milk there.

2. Instead of tipping the bottle all the way up, hold it in a more horizontal position, so just a little bit of milk fills the teat. It doesn't need to be full of milk. There is a common misconception that leaving air in the teat leads to wind in babies. There is no evidence to support this at all, and, in fact, a fast flow of milk out of the baby's control is more likely to cause her difficulties.

3. Once the baby is feeding, watch her and the bottle closely. You need to keep just enough milk in the teat that it's not flowing too quickly, and you need to notice when your baby stops sucking. When she does, you either tip the bottle up in her mouth, so the flow stops, or you remove the bottle altogether and offer it again. Remember how breast milk flows and stops? That's what we're trying to mimic here, alongside respecting your baby's signal that she wants a breather. Feeding actually lowers oxygen saturation, so she needs a break to breathe.

4. This is, of course, a slower way to bottle-feed. From my own experience, it's difficult to do this if you're trying to hold a conversation, eat a meal, drink a cup of tea, or do anything other than intently watch your baby for the full feed. While I

fully agree that parents should be encouraged to make feeding a bonding and enjoyable time where you look deeply into your baby's eyes and take it all in, I'm also a mum of two, who bottle-fed, and I understand that sometimes life happens. If you have a mate over at feeding time, of course, you're not going to be able to pace the feed as well as when it's just you and your baby. If your toddler is screaming at you to put the TV on and the phone is ringing, or the postman knocks on the door, or it's 3 am and you've already been up half an hour expressing, then you are going to find pacing feeds more difficult. But that's okay. This isn't black and white. Pace feeds when you can and be kind to yourself when you can't.

There's another side to this paced-feeding theory. If your baby is used to having a bottle (perhaps because it's been quite a while between you stopping breastfeeding and deciding to relactate), then there isn't really any evidence that suggests that paced feeding helps you return to breastfeeding.

In fact, some IBCLCs I have spoken to while researching this text have said that paced feeding is so slow that it could hinder your attempts to relactate. It impinges on time you should spend feeding your baby, expressing, working on breastfeeding, or getting on with any of the 101 other things that need doing in our daily lives.

On the other hand, I (and some other IBCLCs) are convinced that paced feeding can help you with the emotional and psycological side of returning to breastfeeding. This is because it encourages you to feed your baby in a responsive way. That is, it helps you begin to move away from feeding your baby X amount of milk every Y hours, as is common with bottle-feeding. Instead, it allows you to learn to trust your baby's hunger and fullness cues instead.

One element of relactation that many mothers find challenging is this psychological shift to truly responsive feeding. If paced feeding can begin to help you explore that transition, then it can be helpful.

It's also worth noting that paced feeding doesn't have to be done as described above every time. It could be as simple as you waiting for the baby to take the teat but changing nothing else. Or holding your baby in the more upright position near your breast but keeping everything else the same. Explore the different ways to implement paced feeding and stick with the bits that feel right to you and your baby.

At Breast Supplementer

> *"I broke down and cried happy tears the first time a local*
> *LLL leader showed me how to use an SNS [...] Never*
> *thought it was possible to be so grateful to a length of*
> *plastic tube."* - Lisa Marie

An at breast supplementer (ABS) is essentially a feeding tube taped to your breast near your nipple with a small bottle of milk at the other end. The milk flows through the tubing, and your baby gets milk while suckling at the breast. This assists in building up your milk supply through the stimulation, helps your baby remember how to breastfeed, and can cut down on pumping time if you use it at most or all feeds.

Many mothers say an ABS made all the difference. It saved their breastfeeding relationship, and they are deeply grateful that such a device exists. However, in my experience, it seems that almost as many mothers say they found it far too fiddly and awkward, and quickly disposed of it. That just goes to show that there's no "one rule fits all" approach to successful relactation.

The potential difficulties with an ABS include cleaning the tubing. This can be a nightmare, as it's so thin. Getting the ABS set up and then feeding baby can often feel like it needs about six hands. When I used one, it took both my IBCLC and me to achieve a feed with it. A lot of giggling was involved, because if you can't laugh when there's spilt milk, tubes, and the baby's hands everywhere, then you would possibly cry.

You also need a baby willing to nurse, which isn't guaranteed in the early stages of relactation.

There are two branded devices available to buy, these are called the Medela SNS and the Lact-Aid NursingTrainer™ System. You're looking at a cost of around £30, and shipping that can take a couple of weeks to the UK.

Alternatively, you could make your own, which may be especially helpful if you're not sure you want to purchase a "proper" one in case you don't get on with it.

DIY ABS

This isn't a cheap option due to the need to frequently replace the feeding tube. However, it is cheaper than the commercially available products, and it's an opportunity to test out an at breast supplementor before paying out for one made by a big company.

You're looking at around £3 for a single tube if you buy them off eBay. It's worth mentioning that you can buy cheaper ones from veterinary suppliers. I'm led to believe these are identical to the ones advertised for human use, but I haven't managed to find any information to prove or deny this claim. I am always careful to ensure my NG tubes are specifically for human use. As a parent, you are, of course, welcome to do some more research and make an informed decision regarding this.

IMPORTANT DISCLAIMER:

Nasogastric tubing is not designed to be used in the way described in the following section. Therefore, doing so goes against manufacturer's guidelines and as an IBCLC, I cannot recommend that you use one. There is a woeful lack of research on using NG tubes for lactation purposes so I'm not able to confidently state, with evidence behind me, that a homemade nursing system is definitely safe. Please read all of the information below and, if possible, speak to other people who have used homemade nursing systems before making your own, fully informed decision.

Making a Homemade At Breast Supplementer

Shared with permission from Philippa Pearson Glaze, IBCLC (2018-a).

You Will Need

» An ordinary feeding or storage bottle and teat.

» A 5 or 6 French, 50 cm or 90 cm feeding tube (nasogastric tube).

» A 5 ml or 10 ml syringe for flushing and cleaning the tube—your local pharmacy may sell these or online stores like Amazon sell individually-wrapped sterile syringes.

Setting Up

Slightly enlarge the hole of a bottle teat or vent (with clean scissors) so that you can feed the tubing upwards through the teat. The plastic attachment (an open/close valve) on the feeding tube sits in the milk at the bottom of the bottle (make sure the valve is open). A tight fit for the tube through the bottle nipple will reduce spillage.

Add your expressed breast milk or formula supplement to the bottle. Screw the artificial teat onto the bottle with the feeding tube threaded through it and the valve end of the tube submerged in the milk.

Piercing a second hole in the teat, or using a teat with a vent, allows air into the bottle, so your baby doesn't need to suck harder as the bottle empties. Some mothers find it works well without the extra hole.

Place the bottle on a table close to where you are feeding your baby, or put it in a shirt pocket, between your breasts or between your knees, depending on the length of the tube.

The free-rounded end of the tube should lie alongside the mother's nipple and be taken into the baby's mouth when he begins to suck. Alternatively, you can latch your baby on the breast first, and then slide the tube into the corner of the baby's mouth when you are ready (for example, after he has breastfed on both breasts first).

Some mothers find it useful to tape the tube to their breast with surgical tape or a plaster, and others prefer not to. Experiment to find what works for you. If you tape the tube to your breast before your baby latches, make sure the tape is far enough away from your nipple so that it won't interfere with your baby's latch. Also, check that the tube isn't extended further than your nipple or it may make your baby gag or reach the back of his throat (taping it to the breast will help avoid this). Jack Newman, a Canadian paediatrician and breastfeeding expert, says the tube only needs to be over the baby's gums to work properly (Lactation aid, n.d.; Newman, 2019).

You can alter the flow rate by moving the bottle higher and lower. The higher you hold the bottle, the faster the milk will flow. You might also want to try a 6 French tube instead, as the wider hole will allow a faster flow of milk for a baby who isn't strong enough to suck through the smaller tube.

It's important that the tubing is replaced often because they are tricky to clean properly and, thanks to lack of research, it's safer to guess that they may not handle a lot of sterilising well.

You'll struggle to find a consensus on how often they need to be replaced. Different sources state anywhere from 24 hours to "a few days" if the tube is carefully washed after every use.

Cleaning the DIY ABS

This is lengthy, but thorough and important information.

As at-breast supplementing with a bottle and NG tube is becoming more popular due to social media awareness, important questions have been raised by parents and professionals regarding the appropriate care and cleaning of an NG tube being used in this way. I was surprised and frustrated to discover a lack of coherent and consistent information available for both lactation workers and families around this potentially risky scenario.

With this in mind, I set about attempting to design some guidelines based on the limited information I have managed to pull together from different sources, including NICE, Medela, and manufacturers' information about NG tubes. Here is what I have found.

> **DISCLAIMER:**
>
> NG tubes are not designed with the intention of using them in a homemade at breast-supplementing device. Therefore, using them in this way goes against manufacturers recommendations, and you do so at your own risk. The information in this article is simply to help you make an informed choice about their use.

1. NG tubes are single-use items. This means the manufacturer has designed them with the intention that they will be discarded after they have been used once and therefore, they are **not** designed to be sterilised. Instead, they should be thrown away. This information came about from a telephone conversation with a manufacturer and another telephone conversation with a medical equipment sales rep.

   However, the way NG tubes we use for at-breast supplementing are traditionally placed means that "single-use" equals up to 72 hours if they are being placed nasogastrically, as designed. This is because, once in situ, they aren't being regularly handled, and therefore, not exposed to external dirt and bacteria in the outside environment. The NG tube is then flushed every 6 hours with hot water until it's replaced after 3 days. However, if it is dislodged or removed, then it would be replaced after 24 hours, due to increased exposure to potential pathogens (The National Nurses Nutrition group, 2016; MHRA, 2018).

   This is significant for us, as our intention is to use the NG tube externally at the breast, therefore exposing it to our environment, which is almost certainly a family home with various risk factors floating around such as pets, other children, and varying degrees of personal hygiene.

2. Because NG tubes are designed for single-use, they may quickly begin to break down with cleaning and frequent use. The inside of the tubing can become rough and, therefore, easier for bacteria to adhere to. This then makes effective cleaning more difficult as time goes on.

This can be more, or less of an issue depending on what you're putting through the tube. Breastmilk is safer for longer than formula milk, which should be discarded after just a couple of hours after preparing. Formula is also thicker and may be more difficult to clean out of the tubing.. Some sources recommend keeping an SNS in the fridge in a clean Ziploc bag; the theory here is that if we can keep breastmilk in the fridge for several days, we can keep breastmilk particles we didn't manage to wash away in the fridge for several days too. However, this only works if you've used nothing other than expressed breastmilk (EBM) in the tubing.

Hurrell et al. (2009) found that colonisation of bacteria occurred in 76% of feeding tubes after two days, regardless of whether formula or breastmilk was used in them on a neonatal unit. However, more *Enterobacteriaceae* (which include salmonella and E.coli) were found in the tubes where formula was used.

We should also note that the tubes examined in the study would have been flushed with hot water every six hours, rather than flushed with cold water several times, washed in hot soapy water, and flushed again before being dried and put in the fridge, as is recommended for cleaning a homemade at-breast supplementor.

You should carefully inspect the tubing before each use for any signs of discolouration, kinking, or wear and tear. As soon as you suspect it is breaking down at all, it must be replaced.

Remember that some degradation may be invisible to the human eye, so you might consider discarding the tubing after 72 hours, even if it appears to be okay.

3. Next, we need to consider the baby who is going to be fed with the tube. A premature or sick baby is far less able to tolerate potential contact with pathogens than a thriving, robust 6-month-old. You have got to be especially careful if a baby is considered vulnerable, and I would recommend extreme caution if your baby falls into this category.

4. I touched on hygiene above, but it's an important factor here. If you are ensuring excellent cleanliness of your hands, as well as the surfaces your equipment is coming into contact with, you are reducing the risks of contamination compared to, for example, leaving the tubing lying around near the kitchen sink, where everyone is washing their plates and hands.

The CDC in America changed its guidelines on washing breast pump parts last year after a premature baby died following exposure to bacteria in the sink, where the pump parts were washed. They now recommend that a separate basin is used for washing equipment used for feeding babies, rather than the family washing up bowl.

It is often suggested that you wash parts and bottles in a dishwasher. In fact, some manufacturer instructions tell you it's safe to do so, and this is commonly done. Anecdotally, I found the dishwasher made my parts smell odd and stained them an unattractive orange colour, as well as causing the measures on the side to fade.

There is a recent report published in *Pediatric Experts* claiming that baby bottles and cups should perhaps be hand-washed as the chemicals in the plastic (even if BPA free) can leak, potentially causing health issues later on. The FDA (the Food and Drug Administration in the U. S.) was reviewing the findings of this report in August 2018, but there is no update at the time of writing.

Thorough cleaning of the tubing *as soon as possible* after *every* use is essential. You need to flush the tube with a syringe of cold water at least three times before washing in hot soapy water and flushing again with hot water. You would then spin the tube around to blow out the water droplets, leave it to dry somewhere clean, and then store in a clean Ziploc bag, perhaps in the fridge if we're sticking with the theory that colder is safer.

In summary, due to the single-use nature, NG tubing should be discarded at some point between 24 and 72 hours, depending on signs of visible wear and tear or discolouration. This is essentially irrelevant of whether you are using breastmilk or formula, or how good your hygiene practices are.

Using an NG tube more than once goes against manufacturers recommendations, and while they are designed to cope with 72 hours of use, they would usually be placed nasogastrically and left in situ, which is different to how we use them in our kitchens and living rooms. This means you may prefer to discard sooner rather than later, especially if you are using formula in the tubing.

Once again, I want to emphasise that the information here is to inform only. I'm not recommending you use NG tubes in this way. Whether you do is a personal decision for you to make after doing as much research as possible and speaking to as many professionals as you are able.

I'm proud to be able to end this section with the wise words of an incredible colleague of mine, Johanna Sargeant, IBCLC. Johanna has not only professional experience of using an SNS device but used one herself while breastfeeding:

I fully credit the Supplemental Nursing System (SNS) for enabling me to breastfeed for two and a half years. I had chronic low supply with both my children and while my first ended with grief and heartache at eleven weeks, the discovery of at-breast supplementation for my second baby ensured that I was able to have the breastfeeding relationship that I so longed for. For almost six months, I fed my boy with the SNS. When I first began using this, I was petrified that anyone seeing me use this system would judge me, see me as less than the perfect mother to my children—both the baby I was unable to exclusively feed, and the toddler I was unable to give my full attention to. I was afraid that people might presume when seeing the presence of these tubes that my baby is sick, and the thought of that filled me with panic.

Once I braved feeding in public, though, I began to slowly feel a sense of pride and to see it as my duty to introduce this contraption to the world as simply another way that women can feed their babies—nobody seemed to know about it! I began to experience glimpses of the joy of a breastfeeding relationship: I could bring my baby to my breast when he was unsettled or in pain, and he would find calm there, even with no supplemental milk. I could feed him to sleep and feed him to wake, and when he was 4 months old, I began to be able to feed him throughout the night without any supplement, which was life-changing. Once his solids intake increased, our need for supplemental milk reduced, and I was then able to continue breastfeeding him with only my milk for two and a half years. We did it!

TOP TIPS

While I certainly love and thank this contraption, there were definitely times where I wanted to throw it against a wall and smash it with a sledgehammer. Repeatedly. But I know without any doubt that this contraption is the sole reason why I managed to breastfeed my second for 2.5 years, and for that, I adore it.

So, here are my top tips, as a well-seasoned SNS user:

» Get rid of that cord around your neck. It gets stuck on ears and hair and earrings and everything. It has a plastic "lock" to shorten and lengthen the cord, but that never worked well for me. So, I just got rid of it and tucked it up under my bra-strap or tank top. Easy.

» Get rid of the tape. Sure, you might want to try with the tape for the first 2-3 times to get the hang of it, but goodness, it makes things complicated and makes you feel like you need eight hands. My skin also reacted badly to it within 24 hours. INSTEAD, I would just use a finger to hold it in place temporarily during the latch, and then we were good. Others try to slide the tube in after the baby is latched (though, this never worked for me). There was also no need for tape.

» Get yourself a breastfeeding necklace STAT. Those little hands will be pulling at those tubes constantly, leading to all sorts of issues, so I would manually put my baby's hand around the necklace before latching with the tube, even when he was tiny.

» If you're using formula in there, shake the hell out of it. Ensure there's not a remote chance there will be a minuscule clump that will clog the tube (annnnoyyyyying). If you're using breastmilk, either yours or from a donor, ensure that the milk is warmed enough that the fat is fully melted, for the same reason as above.

» The Process: When Bub was hungry, I'd latch him onto the first breast with no tube, and then get everything ready to go with the SNS for when we switched sides. This ensured that:

> » My heart was coping because I couldn't deal with having my hungry baby wait. Here he was, being latched on and comforted immediately.

> » He was not constantly feeding with the tube. Some babies get used to the tube and won't latch without it. This ensures that this won't happen.

> » He had the chance to just comfort feed and go to sleep if I made a mistake about his level of hunger. 99.5% of the time, he'd start whimpering, pulling at my nipple, and bashing at my breast, so then I'd swap him. The other 0.5% of the time, he would be happy there and just go to sleep.

» I was ensuring that my milk supply was continuing to increase, as I'd only swap him when he signalled that the first breast was "emptied," and he'd worked hard to make more milk there.

Try to remember that using an SNS in public is WONDERFUL! It may be scary but know that you are normalising all different forms of infant feeding, and there were many women that approached me to learn more. For us, this was normal. This is breastfeeding.

Cup Feeding

Cup feeding is used all around the world instead of bottles. Cups are cheap, easy to clean and sterilise, and easy to get hold of. They are sometimes suggested as an alternative to bottle-feeding when the plan is to transition your baby back to breastfeeds. This is because it may avoid the "bottle preference," which can emerge as your baby gets used to the different sucking action needed to feed from a bottle compared to the breast. When a baby is feeding from a cup, he needs to bring his tongue forward, which might help him get used to extending his tongue ready for breastfeeding.

There is a knack to cup feeding, and it's important you do it properly, as there is a risk of causing your baby to choke if you pour the milk into the mouth. They can also be slow and messy for feeding more than small amounts of milk, and some babies might develop a preference to the cup if it's used for a long time. Of course, once your baby is 4-6 months old, you can use a standard open cup, and they can usually self-feed with just a little bit of support from you (and lots of encouragement, because we always want feeding to be bonding and enjoyable).

How to Cup Feed a Baby[1]

Cup feeding is best taught by a demonstration from your experienced health care professional, if possible. Your baby needs to be awake and alert and in an upright position. **Never cup feed a sleepy baby or a baby who is lying flat. And never pour milk into a baby's mouth.**

Use a small cup with a smooth edge such as a medicine cup, sherry glass, or shot glass—your maternity hospital may give you one. You can also buy little plastic cups specially for the purpose, which can be shaped slightly during feeding.

» Half fill or two-thirds fill a cup with slightly warmed breast milk or infant formula

» Ensure your baby is fully awake, alert, and interested in feeding.

» If needed, wrap your baby to prevent him knocking the cup out of your hands.

» Sit your baby in a comfortable, upright position on your *lap*. *You may need a cloth under the baby's chin in case of spillage.*

» Rest the rim of the cup on your baby's lower lip or their lower gum ridge.

» Tip the cup just enough so that milk reaches the rim of the cup. Don't put the cup too far into the baby's mouth.

» Your baby will quickly learn to sip or lap milk from the rim of the cup with his tongue.

» DO NOT pour the milk into his mouth. Go slowly, keeping the milk just at the rim of the cup.

---

1 Reproduced with kind permission from Philippa Pearson-Glaze, IBCLC (2018-b) at breastfeeding.support.com (full article can be found here: https://breastfeeding.support/cup-feeding-newborn/).

» Leave the cup in position when your baby pauses to rest between swallows and is not drinking. Avoid putting pressure on the lower lip.

» Continue to tip the cup enough to keep the milk at the rim of cup.

» Burp the baby, if needed, during the feed.

Finger Feeding (Best taught by a professional)

Finger feeding is where you tape an NG tube filled with milk (like with the SNS) to the pad of your finger and use it to feed your baby. You offer the finger to the baby as you would offer a breast and wait for him to open wide before inserting it into his mouth. You then gently take your finger up to the start of your baby's soft palate and allow him to suckle.

Advantages of finger feeding are that it helps your baby use his oral muscles properly and gets him used to the feeling of your finger at the part of his palate where your nipple should go, and that finger feeding helps babies develop their suck, swallow, breathe pattern used in feeding. The downsides are that it can feel intrusive for some babies, and they might prefer the tube over the breast (Wambach & Riordan, 2016).

Another way of finger feeding is to let your baby suck on your clean finger, pad side up. You then use a dropper in the corner of your baby's mouth to slowly deliver milk. You don't need to squeeze it because the baby sucking will draw milk out and into his mouth.

When you need to refill the dropper, keep your finger in his mouth, squeeze more milk into the dropper, and pop it back into the corner of your baby's mouth. Repeat this until the baby is finished.

Chapter Summary

The techniques in this chapter will hopefully start to transition you and your baby from exclusive bottle-feeding towards at-breast feeds. You might want to try all of them, or you might only want to use one.

If I had to choose only one method to actively encourage, it would be the paced feeding. This is something everyone can do and reminds us that feeding is about connection for both the caregiver and the baby.

A good breastfeeding counsellor or an IBCLC can support you further with all of the feeding methods discussed in this chapter, so do take a look to see what support is available locally if you want some further guidance experimenting with these suggestions.

CHAPTER 5

Making the Breast a Safe Place to Be

> *"One of my boys only began breastfeeding at 19 weeks old [...] Perseverance, lots of skin-to-skin, and just knowing deep down that he would eventually get the hang of it has got us to where we are today, and I'm now rewarded with a baby that gazes adoringly at his mamma each time he feeds. Nothing beats that bond."*
>
> ~ Laura

Some babies will happily return to breastfeeding, especially if the gap between stopping and restarting wasn't long. This chapter is for those babies who need some gentle coaxing to go back to the breast.

Why might a baby refuse to breastfeed? There are lots of reasons, from tongue-tie revision leading to pain, oral aversion from intubation, a negative experience at the breast (such as being pushed and held on by a midwife for the first feeds), a high palate, pain when breastfeeding (birth injury, ear or throat infection, teething pain), oversupply of milk, or—most relevant to us in this book—a low supply of milk.

It's not uncommon for mums beginning relactation to report that their baby simply will not latch at all. Mum offers the breast, the baby arches his back, screams, and refuses to go anywhere near it. This can be so disheartening when all you want to do is get back to breastfeeds. It often feels deeply personal and can bring up feelings of failure, guilt, and shame.

Please know that you are not alone. Your baby absolutely *does* love you. Your body works exactly as it should. And you are a great mother. You must be because here you are, reading a book about how to bring back your milk supply while living in a culture that expects and encourages you to formula-feed.

Skin to Skin

So, with a breast-averse baby, we need to remind her that the breast is firstly, a lovely place to be, and secondly, a place where the milk comes from. This means the very first, gentle, and tentative approach I'm going to encourage you to take is to simply spend time with your baby skin on skin, just like you hopefully had after birth.

As a quick reminder, skin to skin is where you strip baby down to just a nappy, lay back a little, and hold him to your chest, in between your breasts. You can pop a blanket over both of you if it's a bit chilly.

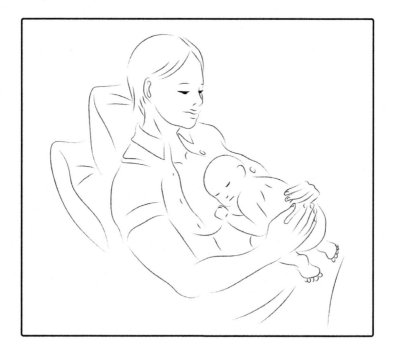

At first glance, this may seem like it has nothing to do with feeding, but actually, skin-to-skin contact (specifically, the baby's chest and belly touching your chest and belly) wakes up all of the inbuilt instincts a baby has for rooting and latching. Such contact begins to remind her about breastfeeding, which she was programmed to do at birth and has likely forgotten as she has adjusted to bottle-feeding instead (Colson, 2019; Gomez et al., 1998; Righard, 1995; Widstrom et al., 1990).

The smell of your body, the sound of your heartbeat, and the way your temperature adjusts to suit her needs help your baby to feel safe and relaxed. Her breathing will calm, and she may well just rest there, enjoying the close contact with the one person she loves and needs most in the whole world (Takahashi et al., 2011).

Over time, this deeply healing connection builds an association with the breast and lovely, warm, safe feelings. For babies who have experienced carers making desperate, flustered, and repeated attempts at pushing them (both literally and figuratively) to breastfeed, this gentle rebuilding of trust and security near the breasts is important.

Sometimes babies don't like skin to skin. If they have spent a lot of time away from close contact, the experience can be overwhelming for them. In that scenario, you should start even more slowly.

You might like to try having his cheek on your bare chest, just for a few minutes. When he is comfortable with that, hold him next to your skin but with a vest between you before even attempting full skin-to-skin contact.

Getting your baby to feel comfortable skin to skin may take a few weeks, or it could take just a few days. Be guided by your instincts and your baby's cues. Never ignore crying and distress.

As with everything in this book, it is important that the experience builds positive feelings for your baby, and not fear or upset. This is because, apart from the mental anguish caused to you and your baby, fear and upset will set you back time and again.

Alyssa Schnell's book, *Breastfeeding Without Birthing*, includes some in-depth suggestions regarding supporting babies to feel supported and safe near the breast before transitioning to breastfeeding. Her work is aimed at adoptive parents and likely traumatised infants. However, it is still relevant for all breast-averse babies, regardless of the trigger.

> *"We used skin-to-skin for Isaac when he was in NICU and not allowed to be breastfed [...] We took it in turns to hold him, so he knew we were there, who we were, and that we loved him."* - Victoria

Co-Bathing

Some babies who protest fiercely at the very idea of skin-to-skin contact seem to relax and enjoy it if they are in a bath with Mum. Co-bathing is such a wonderful and healing practice, but make sure that someone is around to pass the baby to you, and that they are ready with a towel to lift her out of the bath again when you're ready to get out. Babies are slippery when wet and juggling one while you're also wet is a nightmare.

To co-bathe, simply fill a deep bath of safely warm water (no bubbles or heavily scented oils, as you don't want to mask your own body odour, which your baby is naturally drawn to). Climb in and hold your baby snuggly on his front against your body. Ensure his head is near your breasts but also that he is partially covered with the water. Obviously, you want to keep water well away from his face.

Babies often go quiet in the water, perhaps because it reminds them of being in the womb. Some doulas and other birth practitioners even hypothesise that being in water with their mum resets the baby's natural instincts, as it takes them right back to how the womb and the minutes right after birth felt for them. This is sometimes called "rebirthing," and it's quite a fascinating topic if you want to read up on it.

> *"I co-bathed every day with both my babies [...] actually, until they were about 5, and then it became some-thing special they requested until virtually the age of puberty."* - Sammie

Paced Feeding

We have already explored paced bottle-feeding in the chapter above. If you haven't already had a look at that information, now would be a good time to go back to Chapter 4 and have a read.

Paced feeding might be an important part of coaxing a breast-adverse baby to the breast. Holding the baby close to your breast, skin to skin (if the baby is happy to do so), while feeding them is helpful for reminding them that the breast is safe, enjoyable, and where milk comes from.

Of course, feeding your baby against your bare breast may not always feel comfortable for you if you were in public, for example. If this is the case, then there is absolutely no pressure to carry out all feeds this way.

Equally though, if you're happy to feed your baby cheek-to-breast wherever you are, then please do so. Keep on being guided by how you and your baby both feel and stay true to those feelings, as they're essential to everyone feeling calm and connected.

Breast Crawl

> "My first experience of breast crawl was the first day home from the hospital, so about day 3 [...] Just placed my boy skin to skin for some comfort and cuddles, and he started to move. I was so shocked and amazed by this 4 lbs something baby who couldn't even support his head move down my chest, bob his head around, and find his own latch." - Lucy

You may have seen videos of babies breast crawling at birth. It's a powerful instinct they are born with to seek out the breast using many of their innate reflexes. They can see the darkened areola and smell the milk. They kind of wriggle and squirm up from Mum's belly to her chest, where they throw their heads about seeking the sensory stimulation of an erect nipple to latch on to.

Even their hands, which seem to be in the way, help guide the baby to the right landing place over the mum's nipple. The baby will grab at or massage the nipple with her hand, then suck her hand, before letting go, moving the hand away, and eventually latching onto the nipple instead.

This innate behaviour doesn't disappear after the first breastfeed. It hangs around for at least the first several weeks, as it's triggered by the newborn reflexes. A breast crawl, if you have a younger baby, can be a great way of waking up those reflexes, as your baby is taken back to the environment he was designed to be in immediately after birth.

To do this, all you need to do is lean back on a sofa or bed, propped up with pillows, so you're semi-reclining as if you're on a hospital bed. Then you simply hold your baby skin to skin on your belly, just below your breasts. Give your baby time and opportunity to do his thing. This can take up to an hour, as long as your baby isn't distressed. As is the case with all the tips in this book, you should stop if your baby gets upset.

The interesting thing about a breast crawl is that when mums are left alone with their babies, feeling relaxed and confident, they also often show instinctive behaviour to help their baby latch to the breast. She may place a hand on the baby's bottom, move her breast slightly, coo or talk gently to her baby, stroke his skin, and hand express a drop of milk for him to seek out. As soon as we start telling mums to sit up, use a certain position, and shove a boob at their baby's face, it often all starts to get a bit stressful for everyone. So, while you're enjoying this time with your baby, try to relax and follow your instincts as much as you can (Colson, 2019).

I recall doing the breast crawl with Alfie, right at the beginning of our relactation journey. The Breastfeeding Counsellor I had spoken to encouraged me to do this, first of all, to gauge how willing Alfie would be to return to breastfeeding.

To my utter amazement, he wriggled his way up my belly, lunged sideways, opened his mouth, and latched. My milk was pretty much gone, but he stayed there for several seconds while I laughed, and then cried as the awe (and oxytocin) hit me.

That was a pinnacle moment for not only my choice to relactate but for me as a mother. That happened four and a half years ago at the time of writing, but even now, I clearly remember that afternoon and the intense feelings I experienced as my baby fed from my breast after weeks of me denying such an incredible right to both of us.

Babywearing

All over the world and throughout history, mothers have carried babies close to their bodies. It's a natural, safe way to keep your baby feeling secure while also allowing you to get on with whatever tasks you need to complete.

If the baby is happy with skin to skin, this is something you can do topless with a baby in just a nappy. If you're not at the skin-to-skin stage yet, then simply holding your baby close to you in a sling, through layers of clothing, will help. It'll teach him to relax into your heartbeat, breathing, and smell. It will lead him towards associating the breast with safety, which will make latching, when the time comes, easier.

I am not trained to talk about slings and carriers, but there are many "Sling Libraries" in the UK, where a qualified volunteer can talk to you about the best sling for you and your baby. There are many different types so try some on, be taught the necessary safety precautions, and even borrow a sling for a deposit. They are a fabulous resource and should be utilised if possible.

On a related note, I recently supported a mum who figured out how to express while wearing her baby in a sling. The photo she sent me looked complicated, but she was pleased, as her baby was often unsettled unless held. This solution allowed her to pump and meet his need for physical contact.

Here are some words from babywearing and carrying consultant, Kizzy Coll-Cats.[1]

> Infant carrying, close to a mother's body, is something that has been practised throughout history by animals and humans. The use of carrying aids is an old tradition, often created with natural materials enabled ease of movement, prolonged carrying, and an aid to breastfeeding.

---

1   www.calinbleu.com

In Western society, we expect a lot of mothers, and they often have numerous tasks to do alongside caring for and nurturing a child. A soft, supportive wrap or carrier that allows for direct baby- and-mother contact can be a great tool to support the nurture and care of a baby. Research shows that skin to skin improves thermoregulation, regulates the heart rate and respiratory rate, reduces distress, and facilitates self-attachment for breastfeeding. With a soft and supportive sling, which enables direct contact between baby and mother, can, therefore, be used as an aid to offer skin to skin. Even without direct skin to skin the closeness of baby to mother would enable, a number of the benefits to still apply.

Carrying a baby in an upright squatted position close to the mother's chest enables the mother to be close to baby, witnessing and responding to subtle nonverbal communications. The smell and touch of carrying baby close releases oxytocin and provides cues for producing breastmilk and releasing tension in both mother and baby. Some say that having baby close increases babies desire to feed as well as encouraging the mother's milk let-down. A sling can even be used as a feeding aid to reduce strain or to express with discretion while still having baby close. Carrying baby supports the regulation of their circadian rhythm. They therefore sleep better. Babywearing lowers cortisol levels resulting in conservation of energy, can aid digestion and reduces symptoms of reflux as well as supporting the development of muscle strength and motor development through the movement of being carried. This often results in babies who cry less, which also supports the development of parents' confidence. All of these put together are things that aid the breastfeeding relationship. Those who carry are more likely to breastfeed and for longer.

As a new parent, it can be overwhelming; you can find your local babywearing or carrying consultant at www.slingpages.co.uk. Always remember that when carrying your baby. The airway is free of any obstructions and that the chin is off the chest. You feel the carrier is supporting your baby without the need to hold them with your hands. The carrier reaches under the bottom, and ideally from knee to knee.

"My son would cry in the pram, cry in the car seat. Going out was really difficult. Using a sling, though, totally calmed him. He just wanted to be held. He's 2 now, and I miss babywearing." - Laura

Baby Massage

Baby massage is wonderful for both mum and baby. The continuous skin to skin and eye contact trigger oxytocin release, which is great for feeling close and connected to your baby, as well as helping the milk to flow.

Often, babies become quiet and alert during massage. They make intense eye contact with the person giving them the massage and seem to relax deeply. But then, they are all unique, so some might gaze across the room at a totally random and seemingly uninteresting spot.

Babies also tend to go to sleep after a good massage too, which was usually a bonus as far as I was concerned.

In essence, baby massage is yet another opportunity to teach your baby about closeness and skin to skin contact in a way that may feel less intense to them than being right at your breast.

There are countless classes run all over the country. If you're fortunate enough still to have a Children's Centre, you may be able to take a course for free. It's best to go to a course rather than making it up yourself at home. Baby massage is safe, as long as it is taught under the guidance of someone qualified to show you how to do it.

There are also contentious issues around which oil is considered best. In addition, babies shouldn't be massaged soon after immunisations, or if they're premature, newborn, or unwell.

Talk to a local baby massage instructor to find out about their own rules, guidelines, and preferences. Mums often say that they make brilliant friends at a baby massage class too, and the group circle can become as relaxing and healing for the mums (and dads) as it is for the babies.

Here, Kora Lavarello-Monahan from Blossoming Touch shares some lovely words:

Baby Massage: The Power of Touch

Baby Massage is more than just doing something "nice" with your baby. It has many emotional and physiological benefits that not only support your journey as a family but also your feeding and bonding journey.

Massage is a lovely opportunity to practice regular skin to skin and sustained eye contact. as well as stimulating all of babies systems including digestive, immune, respiratory, hormone, circulatory, and the Vagus nerve. The Vagus Nerve activates the parasympathetic nervous system, which calms and relaxes your baby, slowing their heart rate and lowering blood pressure. It also acts as communication, delivering information from gut to brain.

We also know that oxytocin and prolactin work together within the body. When we touch a baby and make eye-contact for longer than 12 seconds, not only do babies release oxytocin (aka "The Love Hormone") helping them feel secure, loved and relaxed, but as a parent, we also release it also. Oxytocin also suppresses the stress hormone cortisol, so when as new parents we are feeling overwhelmed with heightened stress (which is very common as we are learning on the job, often with sleep deprivation!). Massage is a lovely way to recentre and not only calm babies' systems, but also our own. The continued release of oxytocin will encourage bonding between parents and babies. Massaging baby regularly will help parents pick up and understand babies non-verbal cues, which is especially helpful when looking for feeding cues before crying or unsettledness.

Usually, Massage Courses are suitable for babies after 8 weeks. However, this doesn't mean you can't massage your baby beforehand. Gentle containment holds, still touch, and gentle strokes can encourage babies' development and . But it is advised that you do not put oil on your baby for these strokes and keep at a maximum of 5-10 minutes to ensure babies aren't overstimulated. Your baby may not like being undressed, and that's okay. Their skin is sensitive and getting used to the world around them, covering the area that you aren't working on with a blanket, or holding baby close to you can help them feel secure while having a massage.

I appreciate that some of the suggestions in this chapter might seem a bit removed from the work of relactation. I assure you that all of this begins to build a picture for you and your baby—one of comfort, safety, and security at your breast. Babies associate feeding with safety and security, so it makes perfect sense that they won't feed if they don't feel safe. What this chapter teaches you is how to ensure that your baby feels warm and safe, even before you start offering the breast.

All of these skin-to-skin techniques also help your baby to "switch on" their inborn feeding reflexes, which, in turn, allow them to remember how to react instinctively when offered a breast.

Finally, the oxytocin surge you are likely to experience with prolonged skin-to-skin contact will help your milk flow. So, as random as some of these ideas seem, they might help you on your journey.

It's possible that some of these suggestions might not suit you or your baby. That's okay too. Just do what feels good or right to you and discard the rest.

CHAPTER 6

Returning to Breastfeeds

> *"The sheer hard work of pumping every three hours day and night felt completely worth it as I saw the balance of my son's top-up shift from formula to breastmilk."*
>
> ~ Catherine

So, you've been working hard, and finally, you're at the point where you have milk, the baby is latching, and you're ready to reduce the bottles of formula or expressed milk. First of all, CONGRATULATIONS! This is genuinely amazing, and you ought to take a moment to feel proud of yourself.

What follows can feel somewhat crazy, but you're about to enter the world of triple work: expressing, feeding at the breast, and bottle-feeding.

Remember the part about support near the beginning of the book? Go back and read that again because this is the time when you could do with someone to come in and do the washing up for you.

Support aside, how do you begin here? It often feels chaotic and stressful when you know the baby will latch, and you know you have some milk but not quite a full supply yet. I remember almost being paralysed with fear that I might get something wrong, jeopardise my supply, or cause Alfie harm by not feeding him enough.

We'll go over different methods for reducing bottle-feeds here, but before we do that, we need to cover some key points:

1. **Keep pumping.** When babies begin to latch, they may be efficient, or they might need to learn how to feed well. Until you can be confident that your baby is feeding well, it's a good idea to keep pumping after breastfeeding to make sure all the milk has been removed.

   You've probably heard people say pumping isn't an indication of supply. It's a bit different when relactating because you already know your body responds to the pump, and roughly how much you yield each session. So, if you pump right after feeding, you can get a good idea of how much your baby took by seeing how much less milk you express. It can be helpful to know that babies, generally speaking, will take their own individual daily amounts in a range of as little as 570ml for some babies, as high as 900ml for other babies, and the "average" baby taking about 750ml per day. It's important to pay attention to your baby's own cues regarding their needs. (Bonyata, n.d.-b). If you are pumping less than this without offering the breast, then you will need to keep topping up.

2. **Keep a close eye on your baby's nappy output and weight gain.** The easiest way to check whether the baby is coping well with the transition to at-breast feeds is their wet nappy output. Six or more heavy, wet nappies, filled with light-coloured urine, is what we're looking for. Occasionally, it might be just five, but they still should be heavy and light in colour. If nappy output begins to decrease, call a GP or 111 for advice right away.

   Weight gain is the other way we check if the baby is doing well with breastfeeding. We like babies to be gaining at least 30 g a day, on average, until they are 3 months old. Then it's 20 g a day from 3-6 months, and 15 g a day from 6-12 months. Of course, we even this out over a week. It's not usually suggested you weigh your baby daily, as that could end with you feeling somewhat anxious. Have a talk with your Health Visitor (HV) about how often they would like to weigh your baby during this transition process. Once every 2 weeks is usually what's suggested, but every situation is slightly different, so an open discussion with the Health Visitor is the best way forward.

Here in the UK, we don't keep as close an eye on babies as other countries do. If you can persuade your Health Visitor to weigh your baby weekly, that would be reassuring from my point of view.

You can, of course, weigh your baby at home, but be mindful that your scales may not be as accurate. It's always important that your baby is weighed each time on properly calibrated scales, preferably the same set, in the same place as before, to avoid discrepancies. It is natural for weight to fluctuate a bit. Even as adults, we rarely weigh the same each time we get on a set of scales. A change of up to two lines in the baby's red book is usually considered within normal parameters by many health practitioners in the UK. However, a sudden drop in centiles following you beginning relactation should raise some red flags. If this happens, you would be encouraged to reintroduce top-ups and frequent pumping until weight is stable again.

If you're weighing at home and you notice that your baby is moving away from their usual line, it's a good idea to check in with the HV for further support. Ideally, you will have a healthcare provider who is knowledgeable and supportive regarding breastfeeding. It may be that your local, assigned HV isn't always that person. There are private options available in the UK, including hiring an IBCLC or a private Health Visitor, who should be willing and able to work closely with you while you monitor your baby's weight.

During this period, also keep an eye on how the baby is behaving. If you have any concerns (for example, your baby is suddenly sleeping more and is difficult to wake, or won't stop crying), then please speak urgently to a doctor.

As long as you follow these two rules above until you are confident everything is going well, you shouldn't go far wrong. You will protect the supply you have worked so hard to build, and you will be ensuring that the baby is continuing to thrive.

Techniques for Dropping the Bottle Feeds

So, we're protecting milk supply, and we're keeping a close eye on the baby. Now, let's get to the technical stuff. There are several ways of reducing bottle feeds, and you may want to play around with different ones or move through each suggestion as your baby needs less and less of the bottle.

Bottle Sandwich

This is where we sandwich a bottle feed in between breastfeeds. You essentially offer your baby both breasts, and then offer the bottle. Once your baby has had the amount of milk in the bottle, you offer each breast again. As you go along, the goal is to reduce the amount of milk given in the bottle a little bit at a time, say 10 ml per feed, every few days. Or, if your baby is regularly leaving lots of milk, then reduce the amount offered by how much is being refused.

Firstly, work out how many supplements of formula or expressed milk your baby still needs. To do this, let's assume the baby needs a total intake of 750 ml day. Now, let's say that you have been reliably expressing 550 ml a day, you only need to give 200 ml of top-ups (assuming your baby is latching well to the breast, and you are seeing and hearing active swallowing). Divide that 200 ml by eight, which gives you 25 ml per top-up, if giving eight times a day.

Next, you would offer the breast, and let the baby feed, then offer your baby the other breast. Then you feed the baby his 25 ml top-up and express your breasts to ensure he's taken plenty of milk. If your baby appears hungry before his next top-up is due, you would offer the breast again, and use breast compressions to help squeeze more milk into your baby.

If your baby continues to produce his six heavy, wet nappies every 24 hours, and is gaining weight at his (preferably weekly) weigh-in, then you can reduce the amount of supplement by 30 ml a day every few days (so following our example above, we're now giving the baby 170 ml a day, divided by eight, which gives us eight top-ups of a little more than 21 ml each).

Finish at the Breast

Here, you reduce the amount of top-up by a small amount every few days, reducing by only 10 ml for only three of your baby's feeds per day, or no more than 30 ml over 24 hours is often suggested. For the chosen reduced supplement feeds, you would give your baby the bottle as normal but with 10 ml less milk in it than usual, and then you finish the feed at the breast. You would give your baby their usual amount of supplement for all but the three chosen feeds.

If your baby carries on with good wet nappy count, and good weight gain at her regular check-up, then reduce another three feeds by 10 ml. You need to keep expressing until all top-ups are safely stopped.

If you have rebuilt a good milk supply, then this process is probably not right for you, but if you have a baby willing to latch while your supply is still low, then this is an excellent method to use. It will help to increase your supply further while helping the baby get used to breastfeeds again.

Stretched Feeds

Assuming a good milk supply and the baby is latching well, pick a bottle feed to skip and try to only breastfeed until the next time your baby would usually have a bottle. While we don't rely on routines when talking about infant feeding behaviour, you have probably noticed that your baby wants a bottle somewhere around every 2-3 hours, or that she always asks for one at 6 am and 9 am.

Many mothers report that they notice milk supply is often highest first thing in the morning, so you might prefer to start this method with the first feed of the day, or whenever you feel your milk volume is greatest. The baby may well want to breastfeed often during your 2- or 3-hour window. This is okay, and you should follow his cues. Be prepared for cluster feeding (many feeds, spaced closely together).

Switch nursing can come in handy here. That's when you swap breasts every time your baby starts to pull away or fuss. You do this over and over again until the baby is satisfied. It's a great way to increase milk supply.

During the switch, nursing is also a great time to try breast compressions. This is where you apply pressure to the top of your breast with the heel of your hand. You hold that pressure (or compression) and watch as the baby suddenly gets a hit of milk that your hand has squeezed out for him.

Another way to do this is to make a C-shape with your thumb and two or three fingers far back on your breast. You need to avoid altering the shape of the breast near where the baby is latched, so the higher you can get your hand, the better. You then firmly (but not roughly or painfully) squeeze the fingers and thumb towards each other, and again, hold the compression. You'll know it's working because the baby will start to swallow actively and may open his eyes if he was just dozing off.

Keep holding the compression until he stops swallowing, then changes your hand to a slightly different location to squeeze another milk duct. You should only begin a breast compression if the baby is sucking but not swallowing. It's also important not to cause yourself pain.

When your baby stops swallowing, keep moving your hand to new positions until the baby comes away from the breast.

Of course, if the baby becomes distressed and can't be settled with a breastfeed, then you should end the attempt and give your baby a top-up. If this happens, make a note of how long you managed to keep your baby happy with the breast and try to repeat that success the next day.

Once stretching the first feed of the day is going well, you might then either try to skip the second feed or delay it by an hour or so. Simply repeat this until you are at a point that everyone is happy with.

It can also be useful to keep a chart for you to record the amount of expressed milk your baby is taking, the amount of formula she is having, and how much milk you are pumping at each session. It can feel empowering to see that the top-ups are reducing alongside seeing your baby happily stay at the breast for longer.

I want to reiterate that if the baby becomes distressed and won't breastfeed, or you feel uncomfortable or stressed, then it's probably a good idea to offer your baby some of their regular milk in a bottle or however you are supplementing. We don't want anyone to be stressed. It's super important that you follow your baby's cues regarding when he needs a top-up. You will know this far better than anyone else ever will. Trust those instincts and keep a close eye on nappies and weight.

Nipple Shields

If you have a decent supply, but your baby is struggling or unwilling to latch, then you might want to consider using a nipple shield.

That might be surprising to you, as nipple shields can have a bit of a bad reputation. However, in the case of coaxing a baby back to the breast, they can be helpful because they feel similar to a teat on a bottle.

You can also use an ABS(discussed earlier in this book) to preload the shield with milk, so your baby has an "instant reward" of milk as soon as they begin to suckle. You need to ensure that you have the right size shield for your nipples. There are great sizing guides online.

You also need to read carefully the instructions that come with the shields. In addition, express after using them for at least the first couple of weeks to ensure that the baby is removing milk well. It's often helpful to use shields alongside good support from someone trained in breastfeeding.

> *"I began to feed more to drain the breast, and after 20 hours without a bottle, I thought 'okay, I can do this. He doesn't need formula as well.' And we haven't looked back."* - Laura

CHAPTER 7

I Can't Do This Anymore

> *"I'll never forget the pride of feeding her a whole bottle of my own milk for the first time."*
>
> ~ Annie

L et's be straight here; relactation is nearly always both a physical and an emotional battle. As a friend of mine says, "It totally messes with your head."

You want to give your baby your milk. You already likely feel like you failed because of how breastfeeding initially ended, and it's easy to use that to beat yourself up. If you failed once, you'll surely fail again, right? Add in a baby who won't latch, a slow return of milk, and friends who think you've lost your mind, and you have a recipe for feeling like this is impossible and not worth it.

This chapter is a pep talk to help you pull yourself out of your "I can't!" moments. This chapter is *not* an insistence that you carry on if you're confident you are at the end of your journey.

It is not pressure to breastfeed against all odds, and it's not a lecture on why formula-feeding is a failure (because it isn't).

You get to decide at any point that you don't want to relactate anymore, and that is absolutely allowed and okay. There will be no judgment here. I only hope that if you have reached the end of your journey, you can end it in peace and feeling proud of the work you have put in against all odds.

This chapter is much more about giving you a boost if you think you want to stop but aren't sure, or if you're just feeling fed up and deflated.

First of all, take a moment to breathe. You don't need to make any decisions right now. Maybe you've skipped a pumping session, maybe you've skipped several. It's alright. The pumping can wait for as long as you need to collect yourself. If you can, make a cup of tea or hot chocolate. Go and sit in the garden, or on your doorstep, and just exist for 10 minutes. Everything is going to be okay.

Now, consider what has led you to this point. Maybe it's frustration of only seeing tiny drops of milk, maybe it's the heartbreak of pumping for weeks and seeing nothing at all. Is it because your baby is still screaming at you when you try to latch her? Is it because you are just utterly sick of pumping all the time, like some sort of overused dairy cow?

All of these points are covered below, so read what's relevant, take away what resonates, and leave the rest.

"I'm not getting any more milk."

This is so upsetting. You are following the guidelines in this book—pumping eight times a day for at least 15 minutes, using massage, and compressions, and paying careful attention to the pump settings—but still, nothing (or very little) is happening.

Firstly, it can take several weeks to see any change, especially if the gap between breastfeeding has been a long one. When mums induce lactation from scratch (often for adopted babies), it can take a week for the first drop of milk to appear and several more weeks for a full supply to build.

If you have gone longer than a few weeks not breastfeeding, then you may find yourself on par with mums inducing lactation. So, before you throw in the towel, have you been trying long enough to begin to see results? If you're still in week two and you stopped breastfeeding four months ago, you might want to cut yourself some slack and lower your expectations.

This is a slow, often challenging process. It's not an overnight fix. If you aren't sure you're cut out for endless pumping, that's okay. Are you cut out for the next pumping session? The next 24 hours? The next week? How long do you want to try for before deciding to walk away?

Some mums find it helpful to tell themselves, "I'm going to pump eight times a day for (insert number of days or weeks here) and then re-evaluate." Be patient and recognise your fabulous determination and understandable impatience to give your baby the absolute best that you can.

But also remember, you already *are* giving him the best you can. The very act of trying to relactate is such an expression of love and dedication that you should be held up as a super-mum. Take it one moment, one pumping session, and one feed at a time. You will find your own way to the end result that is right for you and your family.

If you've been pumping for many weeks, following the pumping guidelines, having regular skin to skin with your baby, have double-checked that your pump is working correctly, and *still* nothing is happening, then you might want to review the chapter on galactagogues. Take some of the information to your GP and have an open discussion about the risks and benefits of domperidone, or herbal options, such as fenugreek.

"I'm not sure it's worth it."

I'd be lying if I said, "It's definitely worth it!" because, for some families, some mums, some babies, the time requirements for pumping won't be worth it. I don't know what your family situation is like; perhaps you have four children to parent, a business to run, and a partner who is never at home.

It's not my place to decide if this journey is right for you. What I *can* do is tell you what other mums say after they have relactated.

What mums say every single time is, "It was really hard but so worth it." Even those who didn't reach their goal of exclusive breastfeeding will say, "I'm so glad I gave it my best shot because I know I really did try everything."

I've yet to meet a mum who said, "It was awful, I hated it, and I regret doing it." I know my anecdotes aren't scientific, but that's only because relactation is so rarely talked about that no one has bothered to study it yet.

I remember so clearly deciding twice in the eight weeks it took me to get back to breastfeeding that I'd had enough, and I was stopping. Both times, I was certain I was done. But a few hours later, my breast would tingle with a let-down, I'd see the pumped milk in the fridge running low, and I'd look at Alfie and decide to give it one more day before I made up my mind.

This journey is so uniquely personal, and I wouldn't dream of telling you what to do. All I will suggest is that you give it one more day, one more session at the pump, before deciding to stop.

Someone once said to me, "never stop on a bad day," but honestly, there was a time when every day was a bad one, so I don't necessarily buy that theory. Be guided by your own feelings and intuition, though.

If you do stop but change your mind again the next day, or the day after, simply pick back up where you left off; it's not too late.

Some fascinating information I have learned researching this text is that according to a few colleagues of mine, for many women, they reach a low point right before milk production takes a sharp increase. So, if you can find the strength to keep going for four more days, anecdotal evidence suggests you may find things improve significantly.

One teaspoon of breastmilk contains 3,000,000 cells that kill germs. That's just in *one teaspoon*. Breastmilk is like medicine, and one teaspoon a day is beneficial to your baby. I think that's incredible, but it's also relevant to the work of relactation. Spending two hours and more each day attached to a breast pump just to see a few drops of milk each time can be soul-destroying, but those drops combined offer your baby some amazing goodness. It is genuinely the case that every drop counts.

"I haven't got the time to keep pumping."

Someone once said to me, "It's not that you don't have the time to do something; it's more that you aren't making it a priority because it isn't important enough to you." I kind of agree, but, as with most things in life, I think there are areas of grey in amongst that black and white logic.

How badly do you want to make this work? Because if it's important to you, it's amazing how resourceful you can be.

Have you looked into childcare for your older children, or for your baby while you pump? Neighbours, family, or friends may be able to come to your house and offer cuddles, play with the children, or make you a cup of tea.

What about paid childcare: nurseries or childminders? Have you surrendered yourself to ready meals and takeaway, or have you reached out to see if anyone can prepare meals for you? Or hold the baby for you while you do it yourself?

Have you experimented with a battery-operated pump in a rucksack, and a pumping bra so you can walk around the house and use both of your hands?

Have you tried inviting friends to yours instead of going to them, or having an open discussion with them about what you're doing so you can take your pump with you?

There are many, many ways to be creative in order to fit pumping into your daily routine. It could be that some thinking outside of the box is all it takes to find a way that works best for you.

It's also possible that you're single or isolated, have a baby who screams all day long, a potty-training toddler for whom you can't afford childcare, and no money for a one-off takeaway, never mind regular ones to save you cooking. I understand that this may be the case for some of the readers out there, and I'm not here to bully you into carrying on expressing to the detriment of your family or of your mental health.

If relactation isn't going to work for you due to your own unique set of circumstances, then you may grieve or cry. Accepting things that we don't want is often painful. But acceptance can be powerful and healing once those tears have dried.

If you feel that you have no option but to stop, please find a local breastfeeding counsellor or support group and go talk about everything with them. Don't feel that you can't cry about it all, because the crying is where the healing happens.

I want you to know that whatever comes from your attempt at relactation, you are genuinely incredible for even thinking about it. You don't find yourself thinking about relactation on a whim. You do so because you are able to acknowledge the grief you are holding onto about breastfeeding, and because you are driven to do as much as you possibly can for your baby.

When you find yourself at a crossroads, you might find it helpful to step back, pause, and think about all the reasons why you want to do this. The closeness, the convenience of always having the baby's milk with you, the ease of using the breast as a sleep aid, and the feelings of love that it elicits. Write those reasons down. Look at them. Take them in.

Now write down all the reasons you want to stop. Take a good, long, hard look at those too. Are things clearer? Will they look different in another 24 hours? Can you pump for that much longer? Not sure? Do you want to do just one more session and then see how you feel? I'm confident you can because you're a brave and wonderful person to have gotten this far.

But don't just take my word for it. Reach out: get to your support group, talk to a friend, post online, or call a helpline. Get some moral support before you commit to a decision to stop. Talk it out, go over it again and again, write it down, and read other people's experiences. Make sure this feeling isn't fleeting, as they often are. See what tomorrow brings, or tonight, or lunchtime.

All I ask is that, before you stop, you are certain that it's the right choice at the right time. Because if it is—if you are acknowledging and respecting your feelings about this whole situation—then it doesn't matter if your success looks like exclusive breastfeeding or a single drop of milk after six weeks of fighting. It doesn't matter because the peace that comes from a truly informed, well-supported choice is far more powerful than any of the work in this guide.

"I'm pumping lots, but I'm not sure I'm really able to meet my baby's needs."

This is such a common feeling in relactation. When you give a bottle, you know exactly how much milk your baby has taken. You get used to seeing that empty bottle as reassurance that your baby has a full belly. All of a sudden, you've just got your breasts, and they aren't see-through.

For this section, I'm going to assume that you are pumping all, or nearly all, of your baby's daily requirements as discussed further back in the book. I'm also assuming that you have a baby going happily to the breast, doing lots of swallowing, and coming away from the breast (or second breast) content and/or sleepy.

This is a good time to talk some more about responsive feeding, which I touched on in the paced-feeding section. When you have a full milk supply, your body and baby do work in harmony together to ensure that there's plenty of milk. All you have to do is trust both of them to deliver. Which, I know, is much easier said than done when you've had no milk for weeks or months, and you can't quite believe that you've actually relactated.

In light of that, let's go over some normal infant behaviour that might make you feel like it's all going wrong.

1. **The baby wants to feed less than two hours after the last feed.** Frequent feeding is normal. Remember that your breasts meet all of your baby's needs: hunger, thirst, tiredness, pain relief, connection, and reassurance. *Everything* is better with a breastfeed.

   In the final stages of relactation, the baby may also be increasing your supply that last little bit with frequent feeds. This is okay. Look for heavy, wet nappies, a content baby, and some windows of time where the baby goes longer (maybe 2-3 hours) between feeds. Expressing after a breastfeed should also reassure you that your baby has taken the milk you would usually pump.

2. **The baby was sleeping through the night but is now waking up.** This is common, and something mums who have relactated often worry about. Here's the thing, though; it's possible that your baby would have started waking anyway because there are some big growth spurts that seem to result in babies suddenly waking more at night. For many babies, waking well into the second year is normal.

It's also possible that your baby slept longer with a bottle because they were overfeeding and falling into a deeper sleep, a bit like how adults want to sleep after their Christmas dinner.

3. **The baby is fussing in the evening, on and off the breast, but not settling.** This can certainly be scary to the mum who was endured relactation. It's so common that it has a name: cluster feeding.

It's what babies do firstly to tank themselves up before a longer sleep and secondly, to call in more milk during a growth spurt. It can go on for several hours, usually at the same time of day, and it can feel awful. However, as long as your baby feeds well and settles for most of the day. And as long as nappies and weight gain continue to look good, then this is normal baby behaviour.

The good news is that this phase does pass. Sometimes these phases last for days. Sometimes they can go on for longer. Keep looking at the bigger picture and keep offering the breast.

And now, let's look at some reasons you might feel worried about your own body.

4. **Your breasts never feel full.** The early days of engorgement aren't sustainable. Your body hates wasting energy, including on making extra milk that isn't needed. As a result, it slows down production after a few weeks to meet your baby's individual needs with little leftover.

Is your baby happy at the breast? Is she gaining weight? Producing heavy, wet nappies? Can you hear your baby swallowing at the breast? Is she coming away content, perhaps "milk drunk?" Then wonderful, your breasts are doing exactly what you want them to be doing.

5. **You can't feel your let-down.** This is the moment where your milk ducts expand, and oxytocin pushes fast sprays of milk out of your nipple. Some mums feel it, and some do not. Some mums feel it in the early days, but they don't after relactation.

   Look at your baby. You should have noticed a point near the start of the feed where he starts to swallow rhythmically; that is your let-down. You don't have to feel it to have it.

6. **You aren't expressing as much.** Is your baby feeding more at the breast and taking fewer supplements? Then that is more than likely why you aren't expressing it; he's taking it direct from the source, as it were.

   In fact, in the case of relactation, you can express right after a breastfeed to check that your baby has indeed taken a good amount of the milk in your breast. If you usually pump 60 ml, but you find that right after feeding, you can only pump 10 ml, then congratulations! Your baby has taken it himself.

   If your baby isn't producing the six or more heavy, wet nappies we want to see, or is showing faltering growth, then it's possible that you have reduced pumping too early. In this case, you may need to reintroduce some of the sessions you dropped. Make a note to check in with your knowledgeable and breastfeeding-friendly healthcare provider to ensure slow and careful reduction of top-ups and protection of your milk supply.

Remember that babies want to feed at the breast for many, many reasons and, as we aren't mind readers, we need to trust them and our bodies to work together. This can be so difficult following relactation, but as long as you focus on:

» Six or more heavy, wet nappies (and two or more £2 coin-sized dirty nappies in babies younger than 6 weeks) per 24 hours;

» Obvious swallowing at the breast throughout the feed;

» Steady weight gain, tracking your baby's growth curve in their red book; and

» A content baby who is alert when awake and feeds around 8-12 times a day, then you can be reassured that everything is almost certainly working exactly as it should be.

A peer support group, breastfeeding helpline, Health Visitor, or IBCLC can check in with you to confirm that the baby is doing well with responsive breastfeeds.

Final Thoughts

Without a doubt, relactation is hard, time-consuming work that draws toward it many mothers who are initially fuelled by guilt. However, these same mothers are also driven by love and a primal, instinctive urge to breastfeed their babies in a society that doesn't adequately protect and support breastfeeding.

I hope that the information in my book has been helpful to you as you journey along your own path of relactation.

Hopefully, one day, we won't need dedicated information on relactation because women will be supported to meet their breastfeeding goals in the first place. But, for now, at least, it's mostly all in here.

For additional support, you can join the UK Relactation and Adoptive Breastfeeding Support Group on Facebook. We would be happy to welcome you there.

You can also seek individual support through the many avenues of breastfeeding help available in the UK. Peer support groups, breastfeeding cafes, Health Visitor Breastfeeding Champions, breastfeeding counsellors, and IBCLCs are all there to help you on the practical and emotional elements of your journey back to breastfeeding.

And before I go and leave you with the stories of other mothers who have been through this, I want to say:

Good luck, Mama. You've got this!

Lauren's Story

Maddison was born at 36+4 normal but unexpected delivery. She was born with low blood sugars and low temperature. She needed formula top-ups to increase her blood sugars. She latched perfectly and fed well every 2-3 hours, to begin with.

I first suspected that there was an issue at around seven weeks with constant screaming, stomach pain, and being sick after feeds. My husband and I narrowed it down to being a problem with dairy. Within 48 hours of removing dairy from my diet, she started to change, and the symptoms were nowhere near as bad.

At around the four-week mark, she became a completely different baby. At around 12 weeks, she went to feeding hourly day and night, and was not content after feeds. I had her checked for tongue-tie by four different professionals, and they all said it was okay, as she could put her tongue past her bottom lip.

We finally got a referral to the specialist at the hospital, but it was a 12-week wait. We went private and got her seen by a lovely lady who diagnosed her with 70% posterior tongue-tie and silent reflux. All of this had caused a poor latch, and she was unable to transfer milk efficiently, so my milk supply was just dropping at a time.

I then went to feeding every two hours, giving donor milk top-ups and pumping for 15 minutes after every feed. I also requested metoclopramide from my GP. I had to fight to get it prescribed.

It took around three months of doing this before I could produce around 3 oz per pumping session. We then weaned the top-ups down and eventually got back to just solely breastfeeding.

But a month later, I had to have two emergency surgeries that dropped my milk supply again, so we started back with only drops. I was given domperidone this time, and it worked. We are now back to just breastfeeding.

I am due another operation, but I know now that it can be done. As draining as it feels at the time, it is 100% doable and worth every tear along the way.

Sym's Story

When I was pregnant with my first daughter, I knew I wanted to breastfeed. I knew more about it than most mums, so when I ran into trouble, I was surprised.

Surprised that it could happen to me. Surprised it wasn't easy. And surprised by the lack of breastfeeding knowledge in my healthcare professionals.

We struggled with combo-feeding for the first three months, but lack of support meant I soon threw in the towel. I constantly regretted not nursing her myself. I grieved and ached for that lost bond of which I'd dreamed.

After months of sickness and trying every formula on the market, she was diagnosed with CMPA (cow's milk protein allergy). This came at the same time as me seeing a drop of milk on my nipple, so I started wondering if I could get my milk back.

There was very little advice online, but I hired a hospital-grade pump and started pumping every 2-3 hours in the day, and twice between 12-5 am.

It wasn't easy, but the first drops I collected in a bottle were like a gold medal that spurred me on. The first full bottle of breast milk I gave her was my greatest achievement. I swelled with pride.

Slowly, all feeds were replaced by breastmilk. And although I never got her back to the breast directly, I felt amazing knowing she was having the best thing possible.

Jess's Story

My baby was born at 2:19 am. I had been in hospital in labour for three days and was exhausted but elated.

I had immediate skin-to-skin contact, but my baby was not put to the breast. After a few minutes, he was taken to be weighed and cleaned, then placed in a cot in the corner. He remained there for the next two hours while I had stitches and wondered why I didn't have my baby.

Eventually, they tried to latch him on and recorded that he fed for a few minutes, but I don't believe he did. The next time he cried, midwives positioned him to feed, but he didn't latch.

Both of us were pushed and pulled together by seemingly every staff member, and it was decided that I should hand express colostrum and syringe feed. I was helped to hand express throughout the day but not shown how to do it by myself. When the night staff came on, no one came to help me. My baby was getting more distressed, and I had no way to feed him.

Someone attempted to help me hand express but told me I had no milk and offered formula for my baby. It was not my plan, but I didn't feel I had any other option, as I didn't want to starve my baby.

Over the next two days in hospital, the formula he was on increased rapidly and the milk I was expressing was seemingly not enough. I left with a plan to express and top-up.

Over the next few weeks, I saw our local infant feeding specialist, who was unable to find the problem but managed to undermine and patronise me. She then was off work for an operation for ten weeks so advised that I should pump exclusively for that time until she was back and could help.

I found the early days with an unsettled and incredibly refluxy baby very difficult. I was unable to find the time to pump as much as was needed and began to rely on formula more and more.

I was frequently told I was wasting my time, and if he hadn't latched by now, he never would. Friends and family could see the impact pumping was having on my time and so were increasingly telling me to accept that I was unsuccessful at breastfeeding. What they could not see was the impact my failing was having on my mental health.

At six weeks, I read about tongue-tie, which seemed to describe exactly how my baby struggled. I paid privately for him to be assessed, and the practitioner said it was one of the most significant ties she had seen.

However, it did not immediately solve our problems. At this point, my baby was having less than 50% breastmilk, and I was becoming more and more disheartened.

At ten weeks, I attended a La Leche League meeting and was helped by an IBCLC who volunteers with the group. She helped me to position myself, my nipple shields, and my baby, and she got him to feed. Using her tips, I was able to latch him myself almost every time I tried.

I now needed to ensure that I had enough milk to reward his effort. During this time, I reached out to a Facebook group for mums who were relactating. I was supported by the admin and other mums in a similar situation. I was advised to increase the pumping to 8-10 times a day.

I roped in family and explained how important this was to me, and how much support I needed. I cancelled all plans for the foreseeable and stayed at home feeding/pumping as much as possible.

Over the first two weeks, I was able to pump enough to replace two 4 oz bottles of formula with breastmilk. I was still feeding as often as possible and started to find that my baby seemed to be taking a lot more milk at each feeding, so the amount I pumped reduced.

I struggled to be confident that he was having enough milk, so at this point, I was breastfeeding, then pumping, then bottle-feeding whatever I had been able to pump. I was also still giving two bottles of formula a day, but at this point, my husband took over those bottles, giving me chance to power-pump and to sleep.

The first time my baby fed to sleep in my arms, I realised how far I had come and how much we had missed out on in the early days.

I gradually reduced the amount of formula by 1 oz every few days. The baby was being weighed every week, and I had explained to my health visitor what I was doing. I became a bit obsessed by nappy frequency and seemed to be feeding him every chance I got. He had been gaining well, but at one of his weigh-ins, it showed he had lost 40 grams.

I panicked a little over this and was advised to add in an extra pump session and leave it a few days before reducing again.

By 15 weeks, my baby was exclusively fed directly at the breast, with nipple shields. The shields were a faff but felt a small price to pay for the amazing journey we had!

Since that point, we have had various struggles like biting and being too distracted, but in many ways, it's nice to have "normal" feeding issues.

At five months, he took hold of the shield, pulled it off, and began feeding without it, and at around seven months, he gained 4 lbs in a month, bringing him up to the 98th centile!

Lesley's Story

My baby was born by emergency C-section, followed by complications of surgery and a massive blood loss.

We breastfed for the first four days (bar a couple of the wee bottles soon after birth and overnight as I was in theatre and HDU). I was struggling with my own recovery, so despite it going relatively well and having loads of milk, we moved to formula on day 5. One of my main reasons for moving to formula was due to increased lochia while feeding. While rationally, I understood this to be normal and natural, my anxiety was heightened due to a secondary postpartum haemorrhage after my first child.

Once I was properly on the road to recovery—at about 7-8 weeks and following readmission—it started to play on my mind that I had really wanted to breastfeed. I'd had similar issues with recovery with my first baby too.

I noticed when I was getting in the shower one day that I was leaking some milk. After my shower, I used a manual pump and expressed just a small amount of milk. Off I went to Google to see what was possible, and I contacted my friend, who is a breastfeeding peer supporter.

I bought a double-electric pump and starting pumping 6-8 times a day. When I first started, I collected my expressed milk over a week as it helped me to see it build up. I wasn't planning to feed my baby with it anyway, as I was on heavy-duty antibiotics. The first week of collecting, I had 2 oz in the whole week. Then, on one day, I got an ounce, and I was over the moon. Then one day, I tried to get my baby to latch on, and he did! I wasn't sure if he was even getting any milk until I saw the effects in his nappy.

Fast forward another few weeks, and we combination fed. I breast-fed or expressed evening, overnight, and morning, and used formula during the day and just tried not to stress about what he was being fed, and still pumping at least 4 times a day.

Having those special moments where he looked right up into my eyes while feeding, when he rolled his eyes when he rooted for my breast in the middle of the night, they all made the pumping schedule worthwhile. Those times when he was upset and was only soothed by my breast also made it all worthwhile. All of his night feeds were breastfeeds. Those definitely made it worthwhile! It felt like it was the way it was supposed to be, what I had always intended. The fact that he took to it so well just reinforced to me the idea that it was the best for him too.

Between 7 and 23 weeks, we were halfway successful. Over those weeks, we even managed a day or two of exclusively breastfeeding. The rest were a mix of breastfeeding and bottle-feeding expressed milk and formula. At 21 weeks, we moved to mainly expressing (as the baby was becoming less and less settled between feeds), which was still fine, as he was having two of his bottles per day as expressed milk. We were also feeding to sleep, overnight and first thing.

At 23 weeks, he started sleeping more overnight, and my supply was dropping. He used to feed overnight, and I'd hear whopping great gulps, then one day realised that I'd not been hearing him swallow and think he was more using the breast just for comfort, which was still fine.

I was expressing three times a day but getting less milk. He was pulling and chomping my nipples. Basically, between feeding and expressing and weaning—and I also have a 3-year-old—it was time to give up.

I'm so proud of myself for what I've managed but was still in tears at my decision to stop. I'm sure there are loads of other emotions at play here. He's my last baby (not by choice). I was delighted at the joy that the infant feeding team advisors and breastfeeding support group co-ordinator shared with me.

I don't regret moving to formula at 5 days (though I wish someone had suggested maybe just expressing for a few days before really deciding), as it was what I needed to do at the time. However, I'm delighted at how successful our relactation journey was, as it means I won't spend however long wondering what could have been and feeling guilty at not having breastfed for longer.

Acknowledgments

I have been consistently surprised at the willingness of acquaintances, friends, and colleagues to give up their time for me and my book. I couldn't list them all, but a few do need public recognition.

Pamela, who took on the task of confirming my facts and clarifying my rambles with her experience, endless patience, and her wisdom in the field of lactation.

Charlotte, for being the first to go at my jumbled thoughts with her red pen and excellent editing skills.

Jane, who supported me through both relactation and then feeding a breast-refusing newborn; who mentored me practically and emotionally through the IBCLC certification; who stood beside me, held me up, and cheered me on every day, and in every way from the day I first set foot in her peer support group almost six years ago as a new, vulnerable, and isolated mother.

Those who contributed to this book: Kizzy, Maddie, Kora, Philippa, Emma, Victoria, Laine, Johanna, and the mothers who shared snippets of their experiences. Your wisdom and experience are so important, and I'm proud to be able to share it in these pages.

Every one of my friends, acquaintances, and colleagues who didn't tell me to stop complaining about doing the citations, and instead helped me with links to studies and books to allow me to finish this work with my sanity intact.

And, of course, my husband Mike, who never once considered that writing a book about relactation was a poor excuse for shutting myself in a box room while demanding no one disturb me for hours at a time unless it was to bring me coffee.

Notes

The reasons why I stopped breastfeeding:

_____

_____

_____

_____

_____

_____

_____

_____

_____

_____

What I would do differently next time:

_____

_____

_____

_____

_____

_____

_____

_____

_____

_____

_____

The part of breastfeeding I miss the most:

_____

_____

_____

_____

_____

_____

_____

_____

_____

_____

3 reasons I want to relactate:

_____

_____

_____

_____

_____

_____

_____

_____

_____

_____

_____

Who can support me:

_____

_____

_____

_____

_____

My local breastfeeding services can be found:

_____

_____

_____

_____

_____

Ways I can make other areas of my life easier during relactation:

_____

_____

_____

_____

_____

_____

_____

_____

_____

_____

My pumping schedule:

_____

_____

_____

_____

_____

_____

_____

_____

_____

_____

_____

Connection activities my baby and I enjoy: Babywearing/Co-bathing/ skin to skin/baby massage/feeding near the breast:

_____

_____

_____

_____

_____

My relactation goal (e.g. full breastfeeding / one breastfeed a day / 50:50 combi-feeding):

_____

_____

_____

_____

My progress:

Week one

_____

_____

_____

Week two

_____

_____

_____

Week three

_____

_____

_____

Week four

_____

_____

_____

Week five

_____

_____

_____

Week six

_____

_____

_____

References

Academy of Breastfeeding Medicine. (2017). Protocol #8: Human milk storage informationfor home use for full-term infants. Retrieved from: https://abm.memberclicks.net/assets/DOCUMENTS/PROTOCOLS/8-human-milk-storage-protocol-english.pdf

Auerbach, K.G., & Avery J. L. (1980). Relactation: A study of 366 cases. *Pediatrics, 65*(2), 236-242.

Auerbach, K. G. (1990). Sequential and simultaneous breast pumping: A comparison *International Journal of Nursing Studies, 27*(3), 257-265.

Ayton, J.E., Tesch, L., Hansen E. (2019). Women's experiences of ceasing to breastfeed: Australian qualitative study. *British Medical Journal Open, 9*(5):e026234. doi: 10.1136/bmjopen-2018-026234.

Ballard, J.D., & Morrow, L. (2013). Human milk composition: Nutrients and bioactive factors *Pediatric Clinics of North America, 60*(1), 49–74. *doi: 10.1016/j.pcl.2012.10.002*

Bazzano, A., Cenac, L., Brandt, A., Barnett, J., Thibeau, S., & Theall, K.P. (2017). Mothers' experiences with using galactagogues to support lactation: An cross-sectional study. *International Journal of Women's Health, 9,* 105-113.

Bone, K., & Mills, S. (2013). *Principles and practice of phytotherapy* (2nd ed.). London: Churchill Livingstone.

Bonyata, K. (n.d.-a). *Immune factors in human milk*. Retrieved from: https://kellymom.com/nutrition/milk/immunefactors/

Bonyata, K. (n.d.-b). *"I'm not pumping enough milk. What can I do?"* Retrieved from: https://kellymom.com/hot-topics/pumping_decrease/

Businco, L., Bruno, G., & Giampietro P.G. (1999). Prevention and management of food allergy. *Acta Paediatricia Supplement, 88*(430), 104-109.

Center for Disease Control and Prevention (CDC). (2019). *How to keep your breast pump kit clean: The essentials.* Retrieved from: https://www.cdc.gov/healthywater/hygiene/healthychildcare/infantfeeding/breastpump.html

Colson, S.D. (2019). *Biological nurturing: Instinctual breastfeeding.* Amarillo, TX: Praeclarus Press.

Cox, D. B., Owens, R.A., & Hartmann, P.E. (1996). Blood and milk prolactin and the rate of milk synthesis in women. *Experimental Physiology, 81*(6), 207-214.

Cregan, M. D., & Hartmann, P. E. (1999). Computerized breast measurement from conception to weaning: Clinical implications. *Journal of Human Lactation. https://doi.org/10.1177/089033449901500202*

Denis, M., Loras-Duclaux, I., & Lachaux, A. (2011). Cow's milk protein allergy through human milk. *Archives de Pediatrie, 9*(3), 305-312.

Erkul, M., & Efe, E. (2017). Efficacy of breastfeeding on babies' pain during vaccinations. *Breastfeeding Medicine, 12,* 110-115.

Fox, R., McMullen, S., & Newburn, M. (2015). UK women's experiences of breastfeeding and additional breastfeeding support: A qualitative study of Baby Café services. *BMC Pregnancy Childbirth, 15,* 147.

Gov.UK. (2014). *Domperidone: Risk of cardiac side effects.* Retrieved from: https://www.gov.uk/drug-safety-update/ domperidone-risks-of-cardiac-side-effects.

Hauck, F. R., Thompson, J., Tanabe, K. O., Moon, R. Y., & Vennemann, M. M. (2011). Breastfeeding and reduced risk of sudden infant death syndrome: A meta-analysis. *Pediatrics, 128*(1), 103-110.

Hanna, N., Ahmed, K., Anwar, M., Petrova, A., Hiatt, M., & Hegyi, T. (2004). Effect of storage on breast milk antioxidant activity. *Archives of Disease in Childhood, Neonatal Edition, 89*(6), 518-520.

Hurrell, E., Kucerova, E., Loughlin, M., Caubilla-Barron, J., Hilton, A., Armstrong, R., Smith, C., Grant, J., Shoo, S., & Forsythe, S. (2009). Neonatal enteral feeding tubes as loci for colonization by members of the Enterobacteriaceae. *BMC Infectious Diseases, 9, 146,* doi: 10.1186/1471-2334-9-146.

Kramer, M.S., Aboud, F., Mironova, E., Vanilovich, I., Platt, R.W., Matush, L. et al. (2008). Breastfeeding and child cognitive development: new evidence from a large randomized trial. *Archives of General Psychiatry, 65*(5), 578-584.

La Leche League International. (2010). *The womanly art of breastfeeding* (8th ed.). New York: Ballantine Books, 107-108.

Lauwers, J., & Swisher, A. (2015). *Counselling the nursing mother* (6th ed.). Sudbury, MA: Jones & Bartlett Learning.

Leake, R. D., Weitzman, R. E., & Fisher, D. A. (1981). Oxytocin concentrations during the neonatal period. *Biology of the Neonate, 39,* 127–131.

Matthiesen, A. S., Ransjo-Arvidson, A-B, Nissen, E., & Uvnas-Moberg, K. (2001). Postpartum maternal oxytocin release by newborns: Effects of infant hand massage and sucking. *Wiley Online Library (Birth, 28*(1)). Retrieved from: https://doi.org/10.1046/j.1523-536x.2001.00013.x

Mcfadden, A., Gavine, A., Renfrew, M.J., Wade, A., Buchanan, P., Taylor, J.L. et al. (2017). Support for healthy breastfeeding mothers with healthy term babies. *Cochrane Database Systematic Review, 2:* doi: 10. 1002/14651858 CD001141. pub5.

Mohrbacher, N., & Kendall-Tackett, K. (2010). *Breastfeeding made simple* (2nd ed.). Oakland, CA: New Harbinger Publications.

National Health Service. (2016). *Expressing and storing breastmilk.* Retrieved from: https://www.nhs.uk/conditions/pregnancy-and-baby/ expressing-storing-breast-milk/

Neville, M. C., Keller, R., Seacat, J., Lutes, V., Neifert, M., Casey, C., Allen, J., & Archer, P. (1988). Studies in human lactation: Milk volumes in lactating women during the onset of lactation and full lactation. *American Journal of Clinical Nutrition, 48*(6), 1375-1386.

Newman, J. (2019). *Lactation aid.* Retrieved from
https://www.breastfeedinginc.ca/lactation-aid

Noel, G. L., Suh, H.K., & Frantz, A.G. (1974). Prolactin release during nursing and
breast stimulation in postpartum and nonpostpartum subjects. *Journal of
Clinical Endocrinology and Metabolism, 38*(3), 413-423.

Osadchy, A., Moretti, M. E., & Koren, G. (2012). Effect of domperidone on
insufficient lactation in puerperal women: A systematic review and
meta-analysis of randomized controlled trials. *Obstetrics & Gynecology
International,* doi: 10.1155/2012/642893

Ovesen, L., Jakobsen, J., Leth, T., & Reinholdt, J. (1996). The effect of microwave
heating on vitamins B1 and E, and linoleic and linolenic acids, and
immunoglobulins in human milk. *International Journal of Food, Science
and Nutrition, 47*(5), 427-436.

Pearson-Glaze, P. (2018-a). *Homemade supplemental nursing
system.* Retrieved from: https://breastfeeding.support/
homemade-supplemental-nursing-system/

Pearson-Glaze, P. (2018-b). *Cup feeding a newborn.* Retrieved from:
https://breastfeeding.support/cup-feeding-newborn/

Peng, H. F., Yin, T., Yang, L., Wang, C., Chang, Y. C., Jeng, M. J., & Liaw J. J.
(2018). Non-nutritive sucking, oral breast milk, and facilitated tucking
relieve preterm infant pain during heel-stick procedures: A prospective,
randomized controlled trial. *International Journal of Nursing Studies, 77,*
162-170.

Sawadogo, L., & Houdebine, L. M. (1988). Identification of the lactogenic
compound present in beer. *Annales de Biologie Clinique (Paris), 46*(2),
129-134.

Sholapurkar, M. L. (1986). 'Lactare' for improving lactation. *Indian Practitioner,
39,* 1023-1026.

Schnell, A. (2013). *Breastfeeding without birthing.* Amarillo, TX: Praeclarus Press.

Seeman, M. V. (2015). Transient psychosis in women on clomiphene,
bromocriptine, domperidone and related endocrine drugs. *Gynecology &
Endocrinology, 31*(10), 751-754.

Takahashi, Y., Tamakoshi, K., Matsushima, M., & Kawabe, T. (2011). Comparison
of salivary cortisol, heart rate, and oxygen saturation between early skin-to-
skin contact with different initiation and duration times in healthy, full-term
infants. *Early Human Development, 87*(3), 151-157.

Wambach, K., & Riordan, J. (2016). *Breastfeeding and human lactation.* Sudbury,
MA: Jones and Bartlett Learning.

World Health Organization. (2009). *Infant and young child feeding: Model chapter
for textbooks for medical students and allied health professionals, section 2.9.*
Retrieved from: https://www.ncbi.nlm.nih.gov/books/NBK148970